Adult Cardiac Surgery
Nursing Care and Management

Adult Cardiac Surgery Nursing Care and Management

HELEN L INWOOD RGN, DipN, BSc (Hons), MA

Clinical Nurse Specialist
Cardiac Services, North Staffordshire Hospital, Stoke-on-Trent

W
WHURR PUBLISHERS
LONDON AND PHILADELPHIA

© 2002 Whurr Publishers Ltd

First published 2002 by
Whurr Publishers Ltd
19b Compton Terrace, London N1 2UN, England
325 Chestnut Street, Philadelphia PA 19106, USA

Reprinted 2002 and 2004

British Library Cataloguing in Publication Data

A catalogue record for this book is available from the
British Library.

ISBN 1 86156 278 0

Contents

114514

Preface

This book aims to identify the needs of the adult patient recovering from cardiac surgery. It focuses mainly on the more common procedures of coronary artery bypass graft and valve surgery, and provides information to enable evidence-based discussions on the nursing care required to support interventions in the fulfilment of those needs. It is hoped that this text will allow nurses working in cardiac surgery to concentrate on a high basic standard of nursing care, ensuring that the basic needs of the patient are not neglected in the pursuit of technological advancement. It recognises the main complications that may occur and how these can be dealt with.

In discussing the nursing care it is necessary to refer to medical practice and, as more nurses undertake roles traditionally under the remit of medical staff, some of the text may appear medically orientated.

This book aims to answer the questions frequently asked by newly qualified nurses or nurses entering the speciality of cardiac surgery when information about basic nursing care is a priority.

Helen Inwood

Acknowledgements

It would be difficult to list individually the people who have given encouragement and support during the writing of this text, so I offer my thanks to the whole team connected to cardiac services at the North Staffordshire Hospital. Not only are they loyal, they must be the best team in the country. Special mention must go to Mr JM Parmar.

Special thanks must also go to my wonderful family – my husband, children and parents.

CHAPTER 1

Indications for surgery

The last 100 years have witnessed major developments in medicine. Arguably the most dramatic progress has been made in the treatment of cardiac disease. Progressive surgical techniques have allowed for the treatment of most acquired and congenital conditions in addition to injuries caused by trauma. Several cardiac conditions now have a variety of surgical options. Although most surgery in children is performed as a result of congenital conditions, survival rates for some children have led to congenital conditions being treated in adulthood, in addition to the acquired conditions which account for most surgical procedures.

Coronary heart disease

Coronary heart disease is a progressive, chronic atherosclerosis of the coronary arteries and is sometimes referred to as a 'lifestyle disease', because the main causes are related to poor diet, lack of exercise, excessive stress and smoking. In considering when a person may benefit from myocardial revascularisation, surgical advantages should be reviewed against what can be achieved with medical therapy or percutaneous coronary angioplasty or other interventional techniques, i.e. intervascular stents. The timely intervention of surgery is usually for symptom relief or for prognosis.

Angina

Patients with coronary artery disease may complain of angina pectoris – the precordial chest discomfort associated with myocardial ischaemia. It is possible to classify angina states as stable or unstable. The symptoms associated with stable angina are predictable and recurrent, and tend to be consistent in pattern and severity. The classic symptoms are tightness or pressure in the chest, which may radiate to the jaw and/or left arm. Symptoms usually subside within 15 minutes and disappear with rest and/or administration of sublingual glyceryl trinitrate.

On its own, the onset of angina is not an indication for surgery, and symptoms may be controlled over many years with medication. Occasionally, investigation may be necessary to assess the underlying condition of the coronary arteries. Exercise tolerance tests help in assessing the extent of ischaemia. To help in the assessment of angina, and to determine whether there has been any deterioration in symptoms, classification of severity scales has been devised and accepted internationally, but some local modifications may be introduced to ensure objectivity. The Canadian Cardiovascular Society Classification of Angina (see Chapter 2) is frequently used but may also contain criteria relating to everyday activities, e.g. housework. It therefore could bear resemblance to the approach to patient assessment advocated by Roper et al. (1985) with regard to activities of daily living.

Unstable angina

Worsening and increasing frequency of angina attacks may promote a diagnosis of unstable angina. The diagnosis could apply to a mere increase in the frequency of angina attacks, or to a severe episode of prolonged pain occurring at rest, possibly resistant to medical treatment except treatment with opiates. The presenting signs may mimic myocardial infarction without the development of electrocardiograph (ECG) and enzyme changes associated with myocardial infarction.

In these patients, aggressive medical treatment may result in the control of angina but, once stabilised, patients are assessed so that a decision about revascularisation in the form of surgery or percutaneous coronary angioplasty (PTCA) can be made based on clinical and anatomical findings. Patients who have left main stem stenosis, and those who have been on maximal therapy before hospitalisation, should ideally undergo revascularisation during the same hospitalisation. Other anatomical subgroups can be discharged with surgery being performed at a later date but, if these patients become unstable, they can be reallocated on to an urgent or emergency category.

Myocardial infarction

The prognosis and treatment of this medical condition have been greatly affected by the introduction of thrombolysis, coronary angioplasty and bypass grafting, which are proven strategies in improving myocardial oxygen supply.

The concept of PTCA was initially described by Dotter et al. in 1968 when they advocated the use of mechanical force to dilate atherosclerotic vascular obstructions by inserting progressively larger catheters through a stenosed coronary artery. This concept was developed in 1979 when the first angioplasty was performed. Its popularity is largely the result of an acceptable level of success and greater comfort for the patient when compared with coronary artery bypass grafts (CABGs), shorter hospital stay and lower initial cost than surgery. Restenosis of opened vessels is approximately 30% within 6 months. PTCA is considered to be successful when the lumen size is increased by at least 20%, and the systolic pressure gradient between the proximal and distal portion of the affected artery is abolished or significantly reduced. Initially, PTCA was limited to patients with single-vessel disease and proximal discrete lesions. The indications have now widened, resulting partly from operator experience and technical advances. It can be performed on patients with multi-vessel disease and numerous lesions, as well as on patients with stenosed bypass grafts. In acute situations, it can be used along with thrombolytic therapy, although caution is required because of the increased risk of bleeding.

PTCA is performed in a cardiac catheterisation laboratory under local anaesthesia. Surgical standby for PTCA is required in most institutions, because of the possibility of dissection of the artery and subsequent acute coronary occlusion. Surgical intervention is required in 3–5% of PTCA procedures.

Coronary artery bypass grafts

Pioneered in 1969, CABG consists of the construction of new pathways (conduits) between the aorta (or other major arteries) and sections of coronary arteries beyond an obstructed or a stenotic lesion. Table 1.1 identifies the main indications for coronary artery bypass surgery. The saphenous vein is the most widely used conduit.

Repair of left ventricular aneurysm

A left ventricular aneurysm is one of the complications (incidence of 2–5%, depending on the diagnostic criteria) of an acute myocardial infarction, with anterolateral and anteroseptal aneurysms seen more frequently (about 80% of cases) than diaphragmatic or inferior aneurysms (Figure 1.1) (McGoldrick and Purut, 1990). It is thought to

Table 1.1 Indications for coronary artery bypass surgery

Asymptomatic patients	Limited to patients with left main coronary stenosis and those with important triple vessel disease with severe proximal stenosis of a large left anterior descending coronary artery
Patients with chronic stable angina, class I–II	Surgery may be based on left ventricular dysfunction
Patients with chronic stable angina class III–IV	Patients usually have one or more severe proximal stenoses, and have an unsatisfactory response to medical treatment
Patients with unstable angina	Emergency or urgent coronary artery bypass surgery is indicated only when intensive medical management fails to relieve the unstable angina
Patients with acute myocardial infarction	Bypass surgery has little place in the management of most patients with an uncomplicated acute Q-wave myocardial infarction, but non-Q-wave infarctions have the same indications as for unstable angina. Myocardial infarction with haemodynamic deterioration is arguably an indication, but optimal therapy has not yet been defined
Acute complications of coronary angioplasty	Only when there is coexisting acute haemodynamic deterioration is bypass surgery performed immediately after unsuccessful angioplasty
Previous coronary bypass surgery	When a repeat bypass operation is recommended, the indication should be strong, and the patient's general health otherwise should be good

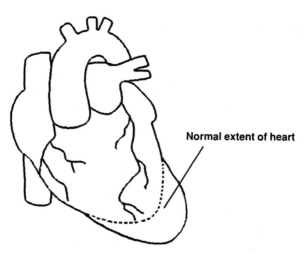

Figure 1.1 A ventricular aneurysm.

occur in muscular areas where the artery has been occluded and where there is an absence of significant collateral circulation. Without treatment, patients generally succumb to congestive cardiac failure or recurring dysrhythmias, and are at risk of thrombus formation in the aneurysm with subsequent embolisation and/or rupture of the ventricle.

Operative mortality rates range from 3% to 30% depending on the patient's age, general status, associated disease and extent of myocardial involvement. The goal of surgical repair is to remove the dysfunctional tissue, while retaining the geometry of the left ventricle as much as possible in order to optimise left ventricular function. Patients often require early postoperative support with an intra-aortic balloon pump.

Repair of a post-infarction ventricular septal defect

Rupture of the ventricular free wall or the interventricular septum is another complication of myocardial infarction originating in the zone of necrotic myocardium. Free wall ruptures, with immediate cardiac tamponade and cardiovascular collapse, are almost uniformly fatal. Ventricular septal ruptures are commonly located in the anterior septum near the apex of the heart and require urgent surgical intervention. Defects may also appear in the inferior septum and the midseptum (Figure 1.2). Post-infarction ventricular septal defects (VSDs) usually occur within 2 weeks of the infarction.

Septal ruptures are rare, but they are often lethal, with a 24% mortality rate in the first 24 hours; they represent the second most important

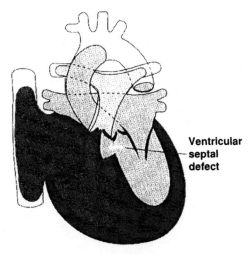

Figure 1.2 Ventricular septal defect after a myocardial infarction.

cause of death after myocardial infarction. Clinical manifestations include pulmonary hypertension, pulmonary oedema and cardiogenic shock. There is an increase in the oxygen content of the blood in the right ventricle and pulmonary artery after septal rupture, because of the left-to-right shunting of oxygenated blood from the left ventricle through the defect into the right ventricle.

Valvular disease

Valvular heart disease, affecting all four of the cardiac valves illustrated in Figure 1.3, can have an acute or chronic presentation. Rheumatic heart disease is the most commonly associated reason for disease of the valves, although the incidence has declined in the Western World over the last few decades. Valve lesions are usually stenotic or regurgitant. Stenosis of a valve produces a pressure load on the chamber immediately proximal to it, so that this chamber eventually hypertrophies. Resultant back pressure on other chambers and vessels may follow. Stenotic valves are usually more life-threatening than regurgitant valves. Regurgitation of a valve produces a volume load, which has an effect distally and proximally. Enlargement of the cardiac chambers follows, with a combination of hypertrophy and dilatation. Regurgitation may be well tolerated initially

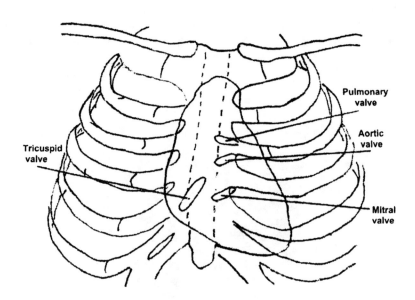

Figure 1.3 Position of the cardiac valves.

because the heart has a considerable reserve, demonstrated by a five- to sevenfold increase in output during exercise.

Aortic stenosis

In this condition, a patient's blood pressure remains within normal limits until a critical stage is reached because pressure is controlled by the baroreceptors in the aortic arch and carotid sinus. A pressure gradient develops across the valve, and it is usually greater than 60 mmHg when a patient presents with symptoms. Stenosis may develop over several years. The left ventricle hypertrophies and eventually dilates. Left atrial pressure becomes elevated, which presents as a tendency to breathlessness on exertion and pulmonary oedema. It carries a mortality rate of 8–9% a year. The most common causes of aortic stenosis are shown in Table 1.2.

It is possible that aortic stenosis can be detected incidentally in asymptomatic patients on routine examination, an ECG or chest radiograph. The symptoms of aortic stenosis develop so insidiously that they are often ascribed to old age. Generally, however, there are three well-known symptoms.

Table 1.2 Causes of aortic stenosis

Rheumatic damage	The cusps thicken and the commissures progressively fuse, producing a rigid valve. It typically presents about 60 years of age and may be accompanied by aortic regurgitation
Bicuspid aortic valve	Although a congenital malformation, this usually presents around 70 years of age. The valve usually functions satisfactorily, although it opens noisily, causing an ejection click and systolic murmur, and eventually stiffening; calcification results in obstruction
Senile calcific aortic stenosis	The valve is usually formed with commissures opened to the annulus, but it is calcified. It typically presents at about 80 years of age. Calcified stenosis is also related to hypercholesterolaemia and patients with underlying atheroma

Effort syncope

On exertion, there is normal vasodilatation in the systemic muscle, but the heart cannot keep pace. This may be the first or only symptom.

Angina

The hypertrophied myocardium becomes ischaemic on exertion, even when the coronary arteries are normal.

Breathlessness on exertion

This is common to nearly all forms of heart and chest disease. The degree of dyspnoea is classified according to the New York classification of dyspnoea (see Chapter 2).

The patient's pulse, heart rhythm and blood pressure are all likely to be normal, but the carotid pulse will slowly rise.

Indications for surgery

The estimated survival for untreated cases of symptomatic aortic stenosis is under 2 years. Those with a pressure gradient over the valve of more than 60 mmHg, even if they are asymptomatic, are at risk and their life expectancy is improved with surgery.

Aortic regurgitation

In this condition, the ventricle has to eject a much greater volume of blood, which is initially achieved by increasing the ejection fraction that can be tolerated well over a number of years. The heart eventually dilates. Filling pressures increase and pulmonary congestion occurs. The main identified causes of aortic regurgitation are listed in Table 1.3.

The symptoms are really non-specific: breathlessness and exercise intolerance. A wide pulse pressure can be seen as a pulsation of the root of the neck, and felt as a collapsing pulse in the brachial arteries. Sudden haemodynamic deterioration occasionally occurs.

Indications for surgery

Some patients tolerate regurgitation for years without symptoms, but surgery is indicated to relieve symptoms of breathlessness and to prevent irrecoverable dilatation of the left ventricle. Surgery carries a better prognosis if it is undertaken before the ventricle dilates.

Mitral stenosis

The left atrial pressure is raised in these patients and increases further on exercise or lying down, both of which increase venous return abruptly. The left atrium is thickened, but not dilated whilst the heart

Table 1.3 The causes of aortic regurgitation

Rheumatic fever	Granulation tissue and scarring produce contracted leaflets with rolled edges. These changes make the valve more susceptible to degeneration from atherosclerosis and calcium deposits
Congenital abnormality	Perforations, prolapsing leaflet
Marfan's syndrome	Chronic or acute regurgitation in an aortic valve with apparently normal leaflets occurs with annular dilatation. This is a generalised connective tissue disorder that weakens the wall of the aorta, producing dilatation and aneurysmal formations on the annulus, the sinuses of Valsalva and/or ascending aorta
Syphilis	This used to be a major cause of aortic root and annular dilatation, but has declined significantly since the introduction of antimicrobial therapy
Trauma	Blunt trauma or extreme muscular exertion which can puncture or perforate leaflets
Reiter's disease	
Ankylosing spondylosis	With the decline of acute rheumatic fever, and a growing population, the predominant cause of aortic stenosis has shifted from inflammatory lesions to degenerative lesions associated with ageing
Endocarditis	This may occur on a structurally normal valve but more often affects rheumatically scarred, congenitally malformed, aortic valves. Staphylococcus aureus is the most common organism. The infectious process more often produces valvular incompetence from destruction of the valve and supporting structures

remains in sinus rhythm. Downstream from the stenosis, the left ventricle is protected and the aorta is characteristically small. Upstream the pulmonary vasculature, the right ventricle, the tricuspid valve, the right atrium and the liver are affected by the raised back pressure.

Patients usually present with pulmonary oedema, often paroxysmal nocturnal dyspnoea, because left atrial pressure exceeds oncotic pressure (about 25 mmHg) so that the pulmonary capillaries and the alveoli can no longer be kept dry. The causes of mitral stenosis are listed in Table 1.4.

Palpitations may be the presenting symptom, but breathlessness on exertion and paroxysmal nocturnal dyspnoea are characteristic. Most patients develop transient or chronic atrial fibrillation as the left atrium dilates and hypertrophies in response to chronic atrial overloading. Thrombus may form in the left atrium and embolise to the brain and lower limbs.

Table 1.4 Causes of mitral stenosis

Endocarditis	The infectious process of bacterial endocarditis attacks the valve leaflets and may extend to the perivalvular tissue. There may be vegetation composed of bacterial colonies, fibrin, white blood cells and red blood cells
Rheumatic fever	A systemic immune process that can be self-limiting, but may lead to progressive valvular deformity. It may be associated with pericarditis and congestive heart failure
Tumour	Left atrial thrombus or tumour, e.g. atrial myxoma may obstruct left ventricular flow

Indications for surgery

As a result of the risk of systemic embolisation, raised left atrial pressures and irreversibly raised pulmonary artery pressures, and for symptom relief, mitral stenosis should be relieved whenever possible; this can occur with the preservation of the natural valve, which carries a good prognosis. Valves are prone to endocarditis; when the destruction of the valve and adjacent tissue is severe, surgery is performed to remove the infected tissue and reconstruct the annulus, so that a prosthetic valve can be securely attached. Surgery to replace a severely deformed, calcified or coexistent regurgitation carries a higher risk.

Mitral regurgitation

This can be distinguished into acute and chronic mitral regurgitation. Chronic valve lesions progress relatively slowly and the cardiovascular system can adapt to cope with a large regurgitant volume. Onset is more sudden if regurgitation is a result of ruptured chordae or papillary muscle, a known complication of myocardial infarction. Acute elevation of the left atrial pressure may cause pulmonary oedema. Causes of mitral regurgitation are listed in Table 1.5.

Table 1.5 Causes of mitral regurgitation

Rheumatic fever	
Floppy valve disease	Also known as mitral valve prolapse, fibroelastic degeneration and infective endocarditis; it is more common in women
Ischaemia	Resulting in chordal or papillary muscle rupture
Endocarditis	May worsen mitral regurgitation

Symptoms are very non-specific, ranging from breathlessness and exercise intolerance in chronic conditions to severe, life-threatening pulmonary oedema. A pansystolic murmur may be present.

Indications for surgery

Chronic regurgitation is generally well tolerated initially (but replacement does not reverse the dilated ventricle), and surgery carries a high risk as a result of pulmonary artery pressures. In acute cases, an operation is life-saving.

Tricuspid stenosis

Rheumatic involvement is very uncommon in tricuspid stenosis. Carcinoid involvement is a rare but a well-known cause.

Tricuspid regurgitation

This is usually part of a multi-valvular disease. Intravenous drug users are particularly prone to endocarditis of the tricuspid valve.

Ebstein's anomaly

Ebstein's anomaly is a congenital disorder of the tricuspid valve that may not require surgical intervention until adulthood. The posterior and often the septal leaflets are adherent and tethered to the right ventricle wall. Although the anterior leaflet is normally attached to the annular ring, all three leaflets are usually malformed. The downward displacement of the posterior and septal leaflets in the right ventricle creates a division of the chamber into a proximal atrialised portion with a thin wall and pressures similar to those of the right atrium. The distal ventricular portion consists mainly of apical and infundibular portions of the ventricle. Tricuspid regurgitation is present and may be mild to severe, depending on the degree of leaflet displacement.

Pulmonary stenosis/regurgitation

This is a rare occurrence in adults but is a common component of congenital malformations, e.g. Fallot's tetralogy.

Endocarditis

Bacterial endocarditis results from an infection on the endocardium by organisms of moderate virulence. The most common infecting organism is *Streptococcus viridans*, which is an inhabitant of the mouth and throat of healthy people. In recent years there has been an increase in infective endocarditis resulting from other organisms, particularly *Streptococcus faecalis*, microaerophilic streptococci and *Staphylococcus* spp.

Infective endocarditis starts on the heart valves, usually the aortic valve, and commonly on valves damaged by rheumatic fever. It may complicate congenital lesions such as VSD, pulmonary and aortic stenosis, patent ductus arteriosus and bicuspid aortic valve, and may develop on artificial valves.

Bacterial endocarditis usually follows transient bacteraemia, which, in turn, may follow dental extraction or filling (*Streptococcus viridans*) or urinary or bowel surgery (*Streptococcus faecalis*). The bacteria settle on the damaged valve and set up an inflammatory reaction, which is followed by deposits of fibrin and the formation of a vegetation that often spreads from the valve to adjacent endocardium.

The most consistent clinical feature is low-grade pyrexia. Increasing malaise, tiredness and breathlessness are common symptoms. After the first week, anaemia develops and the patient begins to lose weight. The fingers may become clubbed. The bacteraemia gives rise to antigen–antibody complexes that cause widespread vascular damage presenting as:

- Osler's nodes – small, tender, red, round areas most commonly seen on pads of fingers and lasting 24–48 hours
- splinter haemorrhages found under the nails
- purpura most commonly observed on the chest and neck

Fragments may break off from the vegetation on the diseased valve, and embolise to produce infarcts in the brain, liver, spleen, intestines or limbs.

The erythrocyte sedimentation rate (ESR) and C-reactive protein (CRP) are always raised and can be used as markers of infection. When suspected, antibiotics should be commenced after a set of blood cultures have been taken. The extent of the infection should be assessed to determine the nature and extent of any surgery required.

Surgery of the thoracic aorta

Surgery on the aorta demands a temporary occlusion. Organs receiving blood from that segment of aorta are deprived of oxygen, nutrients and other metabolic requirements, and specific measures are taken to protect the brain and myocardium from the effects of ischaemia. Lesions of the ascending aorta and aortic arch, which necessitate temporary interruption of cerebral blood flow, carry an increased risk of stroke. When surgery is involved for disorders of the descending thoracic aorta and thoracoabdominal aneurysms, interruption of aortic blood flow between the eighth thoracic (T8) and fourth lumbar (L4) vertebrae can result in paraplegia.

Aortic aneurysm

An aneurysm is a localised or diffuse dilatation of the arterial wall occurring with increasing frequency between the fifth and seventh decades of life. Thoracic aneurysms are characterised by weakening and degeneration of the medial layer, which leads to progressive enlargement of all layers of the vessel. Rupture with exsanguination occurs if untreated. When thoracic aneurysms rupture into the pericardium, death is caused by cardiac tamponade. The standard treatment is the surgical restoration of vascular continuity by replacement of the diseased segment of the aorta with a prosthetic graft.

Aneurysms are commonly described as true or false. True aneurysms involve all three layers of the arterial wall. They can be subdivided into saccular, a localised outpouching from the vessel wall or fusiform, involving circumferential dilatation. Sometimes referred to as pulsating haematoma, false aneurysms are produced when injury to the inner layers causes extravasation of blood through the intimal and medial layers, but the haematoma is contained by the adventitial layer.

Aetiology

Congenital aneurysms are rare. Acquired aneurysms/dissections are associated with medial degeneration, atherosclerosis and trauma. Hypertension is a common finding which can further weaken the aortic wall. They tend to occur in older patients, but patients with inherited connective tissue disorders (e.g. Marfan's syndrome) may develop an aneurysm/dissection at an earlier age.

Aortic dissection

This is a unique condition affecting the aortic media. It is the most common catastrophe involving the aorta. Repeated biomechanical stress, in combination with hypertension and a congenital predisposition, produces an intimal tear, through which blood enters and creates a dissecting haematoma of variable distance within the tunica media. As blood continues to enter the false lumen, it enlarges and impinges on the true lumen. This eventually causes compression of the arterial branches of the aorta.

The 'tear' may originate in any portion of the aorta, but is most often seen in the ascending thoracic aorta, just above the sinus ridge, and in the descending thoracic aorta just distal to the subclavian artery. Severe atherosclerosis of the aortic arch may prevent or halt the progression of any aortic dissection

Classification of aortic dissection was initially described by Debakey and Cooley (1965) and is classified according to the portion of aorta affected:

- Type 1: the intimal tear originates in the ascending aorta, and the dissecting haematoma extends to the descending thoracic aorta or beyond – the 'walking stick' distribution
- Type II: dissection involving the ascending aorta only (the least common, but a feature of Marfan's syndrome)
- Type III: dissection occurs in the descending thoracic aorta and this carries the best prognosis.

This has now been superseded by a more simple classification introduced by Miller (1979). This recognises two types of dissection:

1. Type A (proximal): ascending aorta involved, when surgery is indicated
2. Type B (distal): ascending aorta not involved; usually managed medically.

Both classifications are illustrated in Figure 1.4.

Indications for surgery

Surgery is recommended for all patients with dissection involving the ascending aorta and the transverse aortic arch. Dissection of the descending thoracic aorta is surgically treated when there is continuing enlargement of the vessel, danger of imminent rupture or other complications related to interrupted blood supply. Uncomplicated descending thoracic aortic aneurysms are often treated medically with anti-hypertensives and beta-blocking medications, analgesics, sedatives and rest.

Marfan's syndrome

Patients demonstrate degenerative changes in the elastic fibres of the aortic media and have a characteristic constellation of signs: musculo-

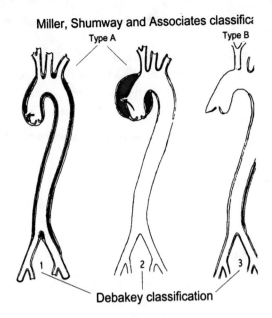

Figure 1.4 Aortic dissection. The top classification is that by Miller, Shumway et al. (1975) and that at the bottom by Debakey (1965).

skeletal characteristics that are the result of skeletal overgrowth, excessive height, kyphoscoliosis, slender long fingers and toes, together with chest wall deformities such as pectus exacavatum or carinatum, weak joint capsules and elongated facial features. Ocular manifestations include exophthalmos, dislocated lens, shallow anterior chamber, detached retina, cataracts and myopia.

Signs and symptoms

Survival and reduced morbidity are dependent on early diagnosis. Pain is a classic symptom. It is often described as ripping, tearing or splitting. It is intense from onset. Abrupt cessation of pain followed by recurrence may signal impending rupture. Compression of recurrent laryngeal nerves can produce voice changes, obstruction of the tracheobronchial tree can cause dyspnoea or cough, and bloody sputum may be a sign of impending rupture.

Surgery for cardiac dysrhythmias

Disorders affecting the electrical activity of the heart produce changes in the rate or rhythm of cardiac impulses. These disorders are commonly divided into those affecting impulse formation, those affecting impulse conduction or a combination of the two. In the late 1960s, operations involving conduction tissue and surrounding structures were devised.

Corrective surgery on the heart itself for underlying dysrhythmias was introduced in 1968, when Sealy and associates surgically divided an abnormal conduction pathway that was producing a tachycardia in a patient with the Wolff–Parkinson–White syndrome. Since then, greater understanding of the anatomical and electrophysiological principles of the conduction system, combined with the development of electrophysiological diagnostic capabilities, has led to the creation of sophisticated devices and procedures to modulate the heart rate, terminate dysrhythmias or ablate the focus of the dysrhythmia.

Surgical considerations

A practical way to categorise disturbances of the rhythm and conduction is to divide them into bradydysrhythmias and tachydysrhythmias, which are supraventricular or ventricular. Determination of their origin is important because treatment and prognosis differ.

Supraventricular dysrhythmias (e.g. sinus tachycardia, atrial fibrillation or premature atrial complexes) originate in the atrium or atrial ventricular junction. Electrophysiologically, these are generally characterised by narrow QRS complexes. Ventricular dysrhythmias (e.g. ventricular tachycardia, premature ventricular complexes or ventricular fibrillation) commonly produce a bizarre (wide) QRS complex.

The tachydysrhythmias are of special concern because they can result in life-threatening symptoms, e.g. hypotension, syncope or pulmonary oedema. Persistent ventricular tachycardia may degenerate into ventricular fibrillation, causing sudden death.

Electrophysiological studies

Electrophysiological testing is an invasive procedure used to diagnose and select treatment modalities for dysrhythmias. Bradycardia and conduction breaks can usually be diagnosed from the bedside ECG but, when there are still doubts, electrophysiological studies should be done.

Electrophysiological studies commonly use programmed electrical stimulation. Preoperative studies are used to assess sinus node function, atrioventricular (AV) conduction and bundle of HIS function, and the mechanism of atrial and ventricular dysrhythmias.

As a result of the serious complications of many dysrhythmic drugs, and their inefficacy in some patients, non-pharmacological therapy has gained increasing attention as an alternative or adjunctive form of therapy. The various forms of treatment include the following:

- Ablation therapy
- Surgical interruption
- Isolation or excision of dysrhythmogenic myocardial tissue
- Implantable defibrillation pacing devices.

Ablation

Endocardial catheter ablation can be performed with direct current, shock radiofrequency energy, laser and cryogenics. These techniques are most often performed in patients with atrioventricular (AV) re-entry tachycardia and ventricular tachycardia.

Supraventricular dysrhythmias

Bradydysrhythmias

Traditionally, temporary and permanent pacemakers have been used for patients with compromised cardiac output caused by profound bradycardia. Pacemakers, introduced in 1958, have evolved from devices that were capable of stimulating a single chamber, to those able to sense and stimulate both atrial and ventricular chambers, adjust rate to physiological demand, provide telemetric information, and autoprogram and reprogram functions and provide anti-tachycardia functions.

Temporary pacing is usually used in an emergency situation, to stabilise a patient with deteriorating haemodynamic function caused by sudden heart block that is related to acute ischaemia or electrolyte imbalance. A permanent pacemaker may be implanted later. Temporary pacing leads are inserted transvenously with a percutaneous method, or leads can be applied externally in the form of adhesive patches.

Permanent pacemakers are indicated for patients with chronic or recurrent severe bradycardia resulting from AV block or sinus node malfunction. A pacemaker system comprises a power supply, housing, leads and an electric circuit. Implantable pacemaker generators usually contain a lithium battery, with the longevity decided by the battery size and capacity, current setting, rate and mode of stimulation. Dual-chamber generators have a shorter lifespan (4–8 years) than single-chamber devices (6–12 years)

Tachydysrhythmias

There are two goals in the surgical treatment of supraventricular tachy-dysrhythmias. The first is to localise the initiating focus or abnormal conduction pathway, and the second to excise, divide or ablate the arrhythmogenic site.

Surgery for Wolff–Parkinson–White syndrome

Dysrhythmias in patients with Wolff–Parkinson–White syndrome are related to the existence of one or more accessory pathways (known as Kent bundles), producing early activation of a part or all of the ventricle by an impulse originating in the sinus node or the atrium.

Surgery for atrial fibrillation

Atrial fibrillation (AF) is the most commonly occurring sustained cardiac dysrhythmia, affecting up to 1% of the general population, 8–17% of patients aged over 60 and up to 79% of patients with mitral disease.

Two fairly encouraging procedures in the treatment of chronic AF include the modified maze procedure and the left atrial isolation procedure. The aim is to eliminate the arrhythmia, maintain sinus node function, maintain AV conduction and restore atrial contraction. This can be achieved by both techniques.

Ventricular dysrhythmias

Ventricular bradycardias may be seen in patients with chronic conduction delay caused by bundle-branch block or fascicular block. Pacemaker implantation is the therapy of choice.

Tachydysrhythmias

The most serious of the ventricular rhythm disturbances are the tachy-dysrhythmias, which may deteriorate into ventricular fibrillation as a result of a primary electrical instability or haemodynamic compromise associated with a rapid heart rate.

Patients undergoing surgical therapy for ventricular rhythm disturbances often have left ventricular dysfunction related to ischaemic heart disease. Ischaemic ventricular tachycardias are commonly the result of re-entrant circuits located in the border region between the myocardial infarction or left ventricular aneurysm and the surrounding normal myocardium. The type of surgery performed will be influenced by the aetiology of the underlying cardiac disease; the surgical approach may be direct or indirect.

Indirect procedures such as coronary artery bypass grafting and valve repair or replacement can be useful in improving myocardial blood flow and cardiac haemodynamics, but they do not destroy or excise the tissue responsible for the dysrhythmia. In patients with a previous myocardial infarction, there may be extensive scarring of the left ventricle and, in some cases, a well-defined ventricular aneurysm. Left ventricular aneurysmectomy has been performed to excise myocardium from which the dysrhythmias were thought to originate. If the dysrhythmogenic site is contained within the resected portion of the aneurysm, the aneurysmectomy could be expected to be curative. However, this procedure is rarely curative because there are usually numerous dysrhythmogenic sites.

Direct surgical procedures to remove the dysrhythmogenic focus fall into two categories: resection and ablation. When these procedures fail to correct the disturbance, termination of the dysrhythmia is achieved with an internal defibrillator.

The major indications for surgery are drug resistance to symptomatic, recurrent, ventricular tachydysrhythmias, drug intolerance or non-compliant patients. Surgical resection or ablation may be contraindicated in patients with severe left ventricular dysfunction. In these patients implantation of an implantable cardioverter defibrillator (ICD) may be the preferred treatment.

Implantable cardioverter defibrillator

Sudden cardiac death affecting more than 450 000 people every year represents a major health problem. Sudden cardiac death is thought to result from ventricular fibrillation (VF) or sustained ventricular tachycardia (VT) that deteriorates into VF. For patients at high risk from sudden cardiac death, anti-dysrhythmic drugs may not provide adequate protection; implantable defibrillators are used to terminate the dysrhythmia.

The difficulty of managing ventricular tachydysrhythmias is related to the fact that electrical countershock is the only treatment for VF. Mirowski (1983) conceived an implantable device that could sense the dysrhythmia and deliver a countershock to terminate it. Initially, defibrillator patches were placed on the ventricle and connected to an internal defibrillator that was activated when it sensed VT or VF. Up to four or five shocks could be delivered per episode of dysrhythmias. Technological advances have produced smaller sophisticated devices that can deliver the defibrillator shocks via transvenously placed leads.

The ICD is prescribed for patients at risk of spontaneous fibrillation or VT unresponsive to pharmacological therapy or when a specific dysrhythmogenic site cannot be located and resected.

Most modern devices are implanted as a normal pacemaker using an anterior left thoracotomy or subxiphoid incision. When surgical implantation is performed in conjunction with other procedures (most commonly myocardial revascularisation), implantation is done through the median sternotomy.

Surgery for adult congenital heart disease

In 1939, the successful ligation by Gross of a persistent ductal shunt between the aorta and the pulmonary artery is often considered the beginning of surgical treatment for congenital malformations of the heart.

Before the introduction of extracorporeal circulatory support, surgical treatment of congenital anomalies was primarily limited to extracardiac lesions, such as patent ductus arteriosus (PDA) and coarctation of the aorta, that could be operated on without the need for supporting systemic circulation.

Improvements in early diagnosis, and perinatal management of congenital disorders, have resulted in enhanced survival for many of these patients. As a result, the number of adults with congenital heart disease has increased and encompasses those who have never undergone palliative or reparative procedures in childhood but who require correction in adulthood, those who have had palliation with or without anticipation of repair, and those who have had surgery and require no further operation.

These patients are also susceptible to acquired cardiac disease and may require surgery for coronary artery disease and valvular dysfunction.

Unlike acquired cardiac disease, which imposes pathological, anatomical and physiological changes on previously normal structures, the major problems associated with congenital disorders of the heart and great vessels are the disturbed haemodynamics and, in some lesions, the hypoxaemia, which result from abnormal morphology, intracardiac shunting and altered pulmonary blood flow.

Why some congenital malformations do not require intervention until later childhood or adulthood is related to the nature of the lesion, the altered volume and pressure loads affecting cardiac function in the neonatal period, and the degree of oxygen saturation of the blood supplying the systemic tissues. Lesions are often categorised as acyanotic (those that do not produce systemic arterial desaturation) or cyanotic (those that produce a bluish discoloration from venous blood entering the arterial circulation and causing atrial oxygen desaturation). Cyanotic lesions can be caused by right-to-left shunts within the heart or aorta (or transposition of the pulmonary artery and the aorta, but usually not in adults).

Patent ductus arteriosus

Patent ductus arteriosus (PDA), seen in Figure 1.5, is the most common cause of left-to-right shunt at the level of the great arteries. As aortic pressure is higher than pulmonary artery pressure throughout the cardiac cycle, shunting occurs in both systole and diastole. This produces a continuous murmur, often described as machinery-like. In addition, the low-resistance pulmonary circulation allows a significant amount of aortic diastolic run-off, resulting in a wide pulse pressure and a bounding arterial pulse. A large PDA will produce a substantial increase in pulmonary blood flow, leading to pulmonary overloading and eventual heart failure.

In adults

A ductus that does not close spontaneously within 2 months of birth usually remains patent. It is also more commonly an isolated anomaly.

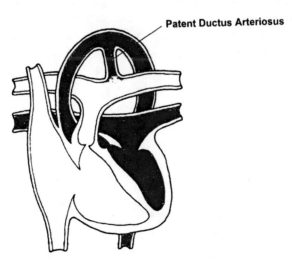

Patent Ductus Arteriosus

Figure 1.5 A patent ductus arteriosus.

Dyspnoea and recurrent respiratory infections are typical presenting symptoms. The presence and severity of symptoms in adults are determined by the size of the PDA, the presence of pulmonary hypertension and the direction of the shunt. Congestive heart failure is a significant cause of death in adult patients with PDA. As progressive pulmonary vascular disease may lead to rapid and irreversible cardiac failure, it is recommended that adults with PDA undergo surgical closure.

Atrial septal defect

Atrial septal defects (ASDs) are among the most common of the congenital malformations seen in adulthood. ASD is commonly the result of a failure in the development of the septum secundum.

Although blood being shunted from the left atrium to the right atrium increases pulmonary blood flow, the right atrium and the lungs are generally able to tolerate this increased volume for many years. This is the result of the distensibility of the atrial wall and the pulmonary vasculature, as well as of the low pressures found within the right side of the heart. Eventually, pulmonary overloading can produce pulmonary hypertension and elevated pulmonary vascular resistance. Pulmonary arterial pressure may begin to approximate systemic arterial pressure, which in turn can lead to a balanced (bidirectional) shunt or to reversal of the shunt whereby higher right-sided pressures create a right-to-left shunt, producing systemic arterial desaturation (cyanosis). With advancing age, patients can also develop cardiomegaly, atrial dysrhythmias, right ventricular hypertrophy and right ventricular failure.

Although bacterial endocarditis is often a risk in patients with congenital heart disease, it is unusual in a patient with an ASD because the relatively large septal defect does not produce a jet lesion that would traumatise the inside of the heart and create a potential site for infection.

Symptoms are usually exertional dyspnoea and fatigue. Initially these complaints may be attributed to coronary artery disease or rheumatic valvular problems rather than to an ASD. The ECG will show some evidence of right ventricular enlargement with characteristically right bundle-branch block in lead V1.

Diagnosis can usually be made with modern echocardiography techniques, showing marked dilatation of pulmonary arteries and an enlarged right ventricle, but cardiac catheterisation may be performed in adults to determine the presence of coronary or valvular heart disease.

Coarctation of the aorta

Coarctation of the aorta, seen in Figure 1.6, is characterised by a localised narrowing of the aortic wall. Abnormally thick medial tissue projects into the lumen of the aorta, forming a shelf, which creates an obstruction to the left ventricular outflow. Blood pressure proximal to the coarctation is elevated whereas blood pressure distal to the lesion is decreased. Upper body hypertension and absent or diminished femoral or pedal pulses may be detected on physical examination.

In adults, the coarctation is often found at the junction of the aortic arch and the descending aorta distal to the left subclavian artery and the ligamentum arteriosum (formerly the PDA). The condition may remain asymptomatic in early life and adolescence. It may present as hypertension, as heart failure (developing between 30 and 40 years old) or as a subarachnoid haemorrhage caused by rupture of a congenital berry aneurysm in the circle of Willis, which is associated in 15% of cases.

Procedures for miscellaneous conditions

Cardiac tumours

Primary tumours originating in the heart and pericardium are rare and occur 10 to 40 times less frequently than metastatic neoplasm involving the heart. The most common cardiac tumour is the myxoma. The aetiol-

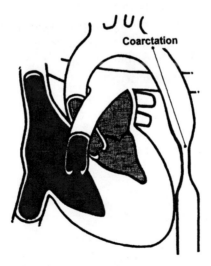

Figure 1.6 Coarctation of the aorta.

ogy of most tumours is obscure, but immunosuppression from drugs or disease, radiotherapy and chemotherapy is one of the exogenous sources that has been implicated.

Many primary tumours are asymptomatic or have clinical features that mimic other cardiac conditions. Patients may have signs and symptoms of congestive heart failure, dyspnoea, othopnoea, elevated venous pressure and peripheral oedema. Dysrhythmias may be present, but the site of origin may not correlate with the site of the lesion. Systemic and/or pulmonary embolism may occur as a result of fragments breaking off from the main tumour mass within the left or right side of the heart. Non-specific findings are common and may include fever, severe weight loss, malaise, weakness, fatigue, arthralgias and skin rash.

In patients with a left atrial myxoma, a heart murmur may be present if the tumour prolapses through the mitral valve. This murmur is often referred to as a tumour plop and may be audible early in the diastolic phase of the cardiac cycle when the tumour falls into the ventricle. These and other tumours may cause symptoms of obstruction and/or insufficiency depending on the size and behaviour of the myxoma.

Chest radiography is often non-specific, although a left atrial myxoma obstructing the mitral valve may produce a pattern similar to that of mitral stenosis. The ECG may show atrial dysrhythmias and various degrees of heart block. Echocardiography has become the most useful non-invasive method of recognising cardiac tumours.

With improvements in diagnostic capabilities, cardiac tumours can be detected early and successfully treated with surgery. Excision of an atrial myxoma is the most common surgical procedure performed for cardiac tumours. Tumours located within the ventricle or the AV conduction system, or attached to the papillary muscles, chordae tendineae and cardiac valves, may also be excised.

Unfortunately, surgery for most malignant tumours is not as effective because of the large mass of cardiac tissue that is often involved, or because of the presence of metastases. Surgery may be performed to confirm a diagnosis and to exclude the possibility of a benign tumour that can be cured.

Atrial myxoma

Atrial myxomas may appear at almost any age, but they occur predominantly in women. Most are benign, although malignant myxoma has been reported. Myxomas are usually located in the left atrium; they are solitary tumours that attach by a stalk or pedicle to the atrial septum, usually in the area of the fossa ovalis. Right atrial, ventricular and mitral valve myxomas are less common. Surgical removal is indicated soon after diagnosis is made, because of the rapid deterioration, danger of embolism and risk of sudden death in these patients.

Myxomas tend to be sporadic, but there may be a familial pattern. Patients with the familial type are more likely to have recurrence of the lesion after surgery; family members may also have myxoma. Syndrome myxoma is associated with the familial pattern; patients tend to be younger and may demonstrate extensive facial freckling. They may have non-cardiac myxoma and endocrine neoplasms.

Pericardial disease

The pericardial sac encloses the heart and consists of parietal and visceral layers between which is approximately 50 ml of lubricating fluid. It is thought that the functions of the pericardium are to stabilise the position of the heart within the chest, reduce friction between the surface of the heart and surrounding tissues, protect the heart against the spread of infection from adjacent structures, prevent cardiac overdilatation, and maintain the normal pressure–volume relationships of the cardiac chambers.

Pericarditis

There are numerous causes of pericarditis. The most common is idiopathic or viral pericarditis; other causes include bacterial infection, malignancy, trauma, irradiation, and inflammation secondary to drug reaction and autoimmune disease. Pericarditis may also occur after recent cardiac surgery. Dressler's syndrome develops after acute myocardial infarction as a result of the body's immunological response to damaged myocardium and pericardium.

Pericardial effusion is a large collection of fluid that impairs the filling of the heart, leading to compromised circulation and tamponade. Pericardotomy can be used to drain the pericardium. With the release of the fluid, a dramatic improvement in systemic blood pressure can be expected.

Constrictive pericarditis

Constrictive pericarditis is produced when chronically inflamed, fibrotic (often calcified), non-compliant pericardium restricts diastolic ventricular filling. The aetiology is often viral, although tuberculosis is becoming an important aetiological factor. Clinically, the patient demonstrates signs and symptoms similar to those of congestive heart failure. The absence of a history of myocardial disease is important in the differential diagnosis. Dyspnoea, fatigue and weight gain are common complaints, and jugular venous distension, peripheral oedema and ascites may be evident. A striking abnormality of constrictive pericarditis, in contrast to the situation with cardiac tamponade, is the failure of intrathoracic pressure changes during respiration to be transmitted to the pericardium and cardiac chambers.

Trauma

Blunt (non-penetrating) injury

Blunt cardiovascular injuries result from external physical forces that create pressure waves on the body tissues. A blast, blunt force or deceleration may produce injuries such as fractured ribs, flail chest, pneumothorax, haemothorax with or without myocardial contusion, or rupture of the cardiac chambers or great vessels. Car crashes, falls and blunt objects striking the victim are the most common causes of blunt trauma.

Blunt injuries do not break the skin, so external evidence of internal injury may be limited to bruises and discoloration of the skin. Injury may result from the direct impact of a force against the skin, deceleration, compression against the chest, upward displacement of blood and abdominal contents, and/or concussion that interferes with cardiac rhythm.

Rupture of the interventricular septum produces an acute left-to-right shunt that is poorly tolerated. Surgical treatment is similar to that for postmyocardial infarction VSD. Valvular injuries often require valve replacement, although reparative techniques are preferred when feasible.

Surgery for injury to the thoracic aorta

Deceleration injuries may cause a tear in the aorta at the isthmus, just distal to the subclavian artery. Creation of a pseudoaneurysm may temporarily tamponade the bleeding. The mechanism of injury and radiographic evidence provide information about the extent of the injury. Superior mediastinal widening, depression of the left main bronchus and deviation of the oesophagus to the right are significant and warrant contrast computed tomography or aortography.

Penetrating injury

Penetrating injuries are caused by bullets, knives, ice picks and other objects that can pierce the skin and underlying structures. The amount of injury is related to the velocity, size and internal movement of the object and the tissue being penetrated. Gunshot wounds are generally more lethal than stab wounds because of the higher velocity and the larger area of tissue destroyed. Acute haemorrhage or tamponade severely compromises haemodynamic stability, leading to shock and acidosis, and the victim often dies before reaching a hospital.

Heart transplantation

Heart transplantation is the procedure of choice for the patient with end-stage heart disease. Recipients are patients who are unlikely to survive more than 1 year and for whom there is no alternative therapy.

Attempts have been made at the development of artificial hearts, and in 1970 a device developed by Robert Jarvik was implanted in calves. The first artificial heart was implanted, in a human, by Dr William de Vries, and the patient survived for 112 days, but in 1989 artificial heart surgery was banned in America. Since then, cardiac assist devices have been developed that can rest cardiac muscle on a temporary basis.

References

Debakey ME, Cooley DA (1965) Surgical management of dissecting aneurysm of the aorta. *J Thorac Cardiovasc Surg* **49**: 364–73.

Dotter CJ, Rosch J, Judkins MP (1968) Cited in Seifert (1994).

McGoldrick J, Purut C (1990) Surgery for the complications of myocardial infarction. *Surgery* 1876–81.

Miller DC (1979) Operative treatment of aortic dissections: experience with 125 patients over a sixteen-year period. *J Thorac Cardiovasc Surg* **78**: 356.

Mirowski M (1983) Management of malignant ventricular tachyarrhythmias with automatic implanted cardioverter–defibrillators. *Modern Concepts Cardiovasc Dis* **52**(8): 41.

Roper N, Logan A, Tierney (1985) *Elements of Nursing*. 2nd edn. Edinburgh: Churchill Livingstone.

Seifert PC (1994) *Cardiac Surgery*. St Louis, MO: Mosby.

Further reading

Treasure T (1990) Surgical correction of valvular heart disease. *Surgery* 1809–16.

CHAPTER 2

Preoperative preparation

Preoperative preparation does not start on admission to a ward before surgery. It starts when investigations commence to assess the degree of cardiac disease. It is important, therefore, that nurses are aware of the various investigations that may occur in the preoperative assessment. Without thorough diagnostic testing, the patient cannot be adequately assessed for risk factors and mortality, which can affect the validity of consent. Once admitted for surgery, the preparation may be regarded as 'routine', although failure to complete this preparation may affect the success of the surgery and have a detrimental effect on nursing care.

The initial diagnosis of heart disease is usually determined by the cardiologist, and is made by reviewing the medical history, a physical examination and different diagnostic techniques to confirm the diagnosis. The medical history and physical examination will also occur on referral to cardiac surgeons, so that an assessment can be made about the extent to which cardiac surgery may relieve symptoms. On admission to hospital, the medical history and some degree of physical examination occur in an attempt to gain a baseline on the physical condition of the patient and, in light of lengthening waiting lists, to determine whether the patient's condition has deteriorated.

Physical examination and patient history

Dyspnoea

This is an abnormal sensation of breathlessness on effort or at rest. With increasing disability, orthopnoea and paroxysmal nocturnal dyspnoea (PND) occur. Pulmonary oedema is not the only cause of a patient waking breathless at night; it can also occur in non-cardiac asthma. A dry nocturnal cough is often a sign of impending PND. In acute pulmonary oedema, pink frothy sputum and streaky haemoptysis occur. With poor left ventricular function, Cheyne–Stokes ventilation makes the patient feel dyspnoeic in the fast cycle phase. Effort tolerance is graded by the New York Heart Association criteria (Table 2.1).

Smoking is a risk factor in heart disease, and any patient should be advised not to smoke. Stopping smoking will not alleviate the heart disease, but it may slow the progression of the disease, improve symptoms, and reduce the risk of mortality and other complications should surgery become indicated.

Palpitations

This is the undue awareness of heart action. The heart rate may be normal or increased, and the rhythm regular or irregular. The sensations may be described as:

- a heavy or pounding heart beat
- fluttering in the chest
- a racing heart (regular or irregular)
- a missed beat
- the heart turning over.

The history of palpitations may range from a few hours to decades; palpitations may occur daily or very infrequently, with intervals of months or

Table 2.1 New York Heart Association classification of dyspnoea

Class	Classification
1	Patients with cardiac disease, but without resulting limitations of physical activity. Ordinary physical activity does not cause breathlessness
2	Patients with cardiac disease resulting in slight limitation of physical activity. They are comfortable at rest. Ordinary physical activity results in dyspnoea (e.g. walking up two flights of stairs, carrying shopping basket, making beds). By limiting physical activity, patients can still lead a normal social life
3	Patients with cardiac disease resulting in marked limitation of physical activity. They are comfortable at rest, but even mild physical activity causes dyspnoea (e.g. walking on the flat). The patient cannot do any shopping or housework
4	Patients with cardiac disease who are unable to do any physical activity without symptoms. Dyspnoea may be present at rest. They are virtually confined to a bed or chair and are totally incapacitated

even years. In most patients, palpitations are not associated with primary heart disease. The patient is aware of a normal heart beat or of simple sinus tachycardia associated with anxiety or extracardiac disease (e.g. infection or thyrotoxicosis).

History of angina

The degree to which angina is suffered and its affect on the patient as an individual may give an indication of the severity of the disease. The Canadian Cardiovascular Society produced a Classification of Angina, which is widely used as a measure (Table 2.2).

Table 2.2 Canadian classification of angina

Grade	Characteristics
I	Ordinary exercise does not cause angina (strenuous activity provokes angina)
II	Slight limitation of ordinary physical activity (climbing more than one flight of stairs and walking uphill)
III	Marked limitation of ordinary physical activity (walking on the level or climbing one flight of stairs provokes angina)
IV	Inability to carry on any physical activity/angina may be present at rest

Syncope

This is the brief loss of consciousness as a result of inadequate blood supply to the brain. The immediate cause is reduced cerebral artery perfusion pressure, which may be the consequence of a fall in cardiac output, peripheral vascular resistance or both. Syncope can occur for a variety of reasons as highlighted in Table 2.3.

Physical examination between attacks may reveal evidence of significant valvular heart disease or cardiac arrhythmia, which gives a clue to the mechanism of syncope. The lying and standing blood pressure should be checked as a matter of course, but the absence of a falling blood pressure on standing does not rule out the presence of orthostatic hypotension.

Cyanosis

Central cyanosis should be detectable when arterial saturation is less than 85% and when there is more than 5 g of reduced haemoglobin present. It is more difficult to detect if the patient is anaemic. Cardiac cyanosis is the result of inadequate uptake of oxygen in the lungs secondary to pulmonary disease, or of right-to-left shunting, which results in deoxygenated blood bypassing the lungs and passing directly into the systemic

Table 2.3 Causes of syncope

Cause	Contributing factors
Inappropriate vasodilatation	Simple vasovagal faint
	Malignant vasovagal syndrome
	Hypersensitive carotid sinus syndrome
	Micturition syncope
	Orthostatic hypotension (diabetes/Parkinson's disease, age)
	Hypotensive drugs
Impaired cardiac function	Extreme bradycardia (heart block, sinoatrial disorder)
	Paroxysmal tachycardia
	Myocardial ischaemia
Obstruction to ventricular emptying	Aortic stenosis
	Hypertrophic obstructive cardiomyopathy
	Pulmonary stenosis
	Pulmonary hypertension
Reduced ventricular filling	Cough syncope
	Micturition syncope
	Atrial myxoma
	Ball-valve thrombus of atrium
	Pulmonary embolism
Hypovolaemia	Excessive diuretic therapy
	Haemorrhage

circulation. It is characterised by cyanosis, which affects the mouth and tongue as well as the extremities – these are warm to the touch.

Peripheral cyanosis in the absence of central cyanosis may be caused by peripheral vasoconstriction and stagnation of the blood in the capillaries. It is best seen in the extremities and the lips, and is often associated with coldness of the part. It may occur in heart failure or be the result of local causes.

Embolism

Both systemic and pulmonary embolism are common in cardiac disease. The following are some of the common factors:

* atrial fibrillation
* aortic stenosis
* mitral stenosis
* infective endocarditis
* left atrial myxoma.

Oedema

Factors important in cardiac disease are elevated venous pressure (congestive cardiac failure, pericardial constriction), increased extracellular volume (salt and water retention), secondary hyperaldosteronism, hypoalbuminaemia (liver congestion, anorexia and poor diet), venous disease and secondary renal failure.

Acute oedema and ascites may develop in pericardial constriction. Protein-losing enteropathy can occur with a prolonged high venous pressure exacerbating oedema. Patients presenting with pulmonary oedema in the preoperative period could be commenced on a short course of diuretics, but the identification of pulmonary oedema immediately preoperatively does not exclude the patient from surgery.

Physical examination

The physical examination should start with the hands, because they can indicate the extent of the disease as well as the type of disease. Table 2.4 demonstrates some of the manifestations seen on the hands in the presence of cardiac disease.

Table 2.4 The appearance of hands in cardiac disease

Appearance of hands	Underlying disease
Dilated hands	Carbon dioxide retention
Cold hands Peripheral cyanosis	Poor flows, hyperdynamic circulation
Clubbing	Cyanotic congenital heart disease, infective endocarditis
Capillary pulsation	Aortic regurgitation, patent ductus arteriosus
Osler's nodes, Janeway lesions, splinter haemorrhages	Infective endocarditis
Nail-fold telangiectases	Collagen vascular disease
Arachnodactyly	Marfan's syndrome
Polydactyly, syndactyly, triphalangeal thumbs	Atrial septal defect

Coldness of the extremities is the result of vasoconstriction or obstruction of the superficial blood vessels, so that the blood supply to the skin is reduced. In heart disease, it is often caused by the peripheral vasoconstriction that follows a fall in cardiac output. In conditions with a high cardiac output, the peripheral vessels are dilated and the skin is very warm.

Facial and general appearance

- Down's syndrome: an atrioventricular canal defect, which is a complicated and serious malformation; it occurs within 7 weeks of foetal life and is basically a malformation of the septum giving rise to a large VSD or ASD
- Elf-like faces: supravalvular aortic stenosis
- Turner's syndrome: coarctation, aortic stenosis
- Moon-like plump faces: pulmonary stenosis
- Noonan's syndrome: pulmonary stenosis, peripheral pulmonary artery stenosis
- Mitral facies with pulmonary hypertension
- Central cyanosis
- Differential cyanosis in patent ductus arteriosus (PDA) with pulmonary hypertension or interrupted aortic arch
- Xanthelasma.

Teeth must be checked as part of the general cardiovascular examination. The condition of the mouth and teeth is particularly important in patients prone to bacterial endocarditis and under review for valvular surgery. In most cases, valve surgery will not occur until the patient has undergone a full dental screening for tooth decay. In many cases, this results in patients having a tooth/teeth extraction before surgery. Patients should undergo regular check-ups (patients who attend the dentist at regular intervals, i.e. 6-monthly, will not require dental screening before surgery, unless the patient is aware of tooth decay that has not been treated). It is also important to note the presence of dentures, caps and crowns. Although this has no impact on surgery, it is important for anaesthesia and placement of the endotracheal tube.

The pulse

The pulse rate and rhythm should be determined by feeling the radial pulse, and certain characteristics of the pulse may be indicative of heart disease. The pulse volume is dependent on the pulse pressure. A small pulse volume indicates a small stroke volume, and is often associated with peripheral vasoconstriction or severe heart disease. A large pulse volume is associated with a large stroke volume and a low peripheral resistance.

The pulse wave, felt at the carotid artery, is also helpful in diagnosis. The collapsing pulse (water-hammer pulse) is associated most strongly with aortic incompetence, but it may also be present in PDA or a rigid atherosclerotic aorta. A plateau pulse is found in severe aortic stenosis. Pulsus bisferiens is found in patients with a combined aortic stenosis and regurgitation or in pure aortic regurgitation. Pulsus alternans is found in left ventricular failure, and pulsus paradoxus in constrictive pericarditis and pericardial effusions.

The neck veins should be examined in the recumbent patient with the head and shoulders raised 30° from the horizontal. At this angle, the column of blood in the jugular system should reach the level of the clavicle. Raised jugular pressure is found in heart failure and in certain conditions associated with a high cardiac output.

Blood pressure measurements are important in relation to determining hypertension. Subclavian artery stenosis, which may be identified by differential arm blood pressure between the two arms, i.e. the differing blood pressure of each arm, could be a contraindication to the use of pedicled internal mammary grafts.

Percussion of the heart

This percussion may provide a crude estimate of heart size, but a radiograph is much more accurate. It may have a place in the diagnosis of pericardial effusion when the area of cardiac dullness is extended to the right of the sternum and to the second intercostal space.

Auscultation: heart sounds and murmurs

Vibrations within the heart are of sufficient volume to be heard through a stethoscope. If the noise is brief, it is a heart sound. A more prolonged sound is a murmur. For accurate auscultation, the stethoscope used should have tubing no longer than 30 cm, and have both a diaphragm and a bell ear piece.

Murmurs result from vibrations created by turbulent blood flow. Turbulence is encouraged by reduced blood viscosity, high velocity flow, and an abrupt change in the calibre of a vessel or chamber.

The presence of a heart murmur may warrant preoperative echocardiography if a non-valvular abnormality has been identified at cardiac catheterisation. The new onset of ischaemic mitral regurgitation or unsuspected aortic valve disease may occasionally be detected.

Investigations

Many investigations are available to aid in the diagnosis of cardiac disease and will allow the severity of the disease to be risk stratified, i.e. determination of the risk to the patient of further acute episodes without medical or surgical invasive intervention. These investigations may be invasive or non-invasive and available at either every hospital or a few specialised centres.

Electrocardiograph

The electrocardiograph (ECG) is the most widely used method of cardiac assessment. A resting 12-lead ECG provides baseline information about the electrical activity of the heart. It can detect abnormal cardiac rhythms, conduction defects, and signs of ischaemia (ST segment changes) or infarction (Q waves); it also provides information about the position of the heart and the size of the cardiac chambers. Results of the ECG are correlated to clinical data obtained from the history and physical examination.

The ECG may be normal at rest in the presence of coronary artery disease, with abnormal changes becoming apparent only with exercise. These patients may undergo continuous ECG with a Holter monitor.

Exercise ECG

After myocardial infarction (MI), the prognosis of the patient is very dependent on left ventricular function, which is reflected in an exercise test using workload and blood pressure. An exercise test can be safely carried out 7–10 days after an MI. Exercise ECG can predict the risk of a future serious cardiac event, including non-fatal MI and cardiac death. This is important in deciding who should have coronary angiography and, subsequently, who should be considered for revascularisation. Patients walk on a gradually inclining treadmill until they reach a target heart rate or demonstrate symptoms of hypertension, ventricular dysrhythmias, ST segment changes or chest pain.

Exercise testing has two main aims:

1. To provoke a symptom (usually chest pain or dyspnoea) or a specific ECG abnormality (usually ST-segment depression) by increasing cardiac work
2. To determine the workload achieved at the time of the response or maximum effort.

A crude method of calculating the prognosis for coronary artery disease is based on ST depression and exercise time, which allows for half of all patients to be classified as high or low risk. The results also provide some indication of the patient's functional status. As waiting lists for surgery continue to lengthen, exercise tests can be a useful aid in determining urgency, but current resources prevent it from being used routinely for this purpose.

Diagnosis of coronary heart disease as a result of exercise testing

ST depression during exercise testing

There is no absolute criterion for the diagnosis of coronary artery disease by exercise testing. ST depression does not occur during or immediately after exercise in all patients who have been proved to have coronary artery disease by angiography; conversely, it does develop in a few patients with normal coronary arteries. The diagnostic sensitivity of ST-segment depression for the presence of coronary artery disease varies from 50% to 90%. The percentage is higher in multivessel disease, and lower in single-vessel disease, with an overall average of 66% (Dargie, 1993).

Various features, in addition to ST depression, may occur during exercise testing and may help in the overall evaluation of a patient with suspected ischaemic heart disease.

The presenting symptom

The development of the discomfort with which the patient presents is useful, especially in the absence of ST-segment depression. Failure of the presenting symptom to occur does not detract from the diagnostic value of ST segment depression.

Blood pressure

A rise in systolic pressure of less than 120 mmHg or a fall of more than or equal to 10 mmHg may be the result of medication. Clinical judgement is required, but it is safer to regard these features as indicating severe ischaemia or poor left ventricular function until clarified by further tests. ST elevation in a patient with a previous Q wave MI usually indicates an underlying dyskinetic segment. In the absence of Q waves, ST elevation indicates severe ischaemia.

Pseudonormalisation, in which a previously inverted T wave or depressed ST segment normalises during exercise, is a subtle but less reliable marker for myocardial revascularisation.

Arrhythmia

If ventricular ectopic activity appears or increases, underlying myocardial ischaemia or left ventricular dysfunction should be suspected.

Exercise testing can provide an objective assessment of both the severity of symptoms and the degree of limitation imposed by cardiac or other disease (functional capacity). With heart failure, cardiac output at rest is preserved until cardiac dysfunction is advanced; measurement of exercise capacity is a valuable method of measuring cardiac reserve.

The Bruce Treadmill protocol, or one of its modifications, is used by most centres in the UK.

Exercise ECG can classify patients into those at high, medium or low risk of having, or developing, a serious complication of coronary heart disease. Greater definition of diagnosis or risk requires further investigation of ventricular function, myocardial perfusion or coronary anatomy by radionuclide tests, echocardiography and coronary angiography.

Exercise testing may be useful in some patients after drug therapy, rehabilitation, revascularisation, pacemaker implantation or cardiac transplant. It is unreliable in predicting the presence or development of restenosis of patent or blocked coronary artery bypass grafts. It is useful in evaluating the immediate or late success of the procedure in terms of improved exercise capacity or ECG evidence of reversible ischaemia.

Radiography

Posteroanterior (PA) and lateral chest radiographs provide important information about the size of the heart, thoracic aorta and pulmonary vasculature, including signs of pulmonary artery or pulmonary venous hypertension. Signs of pulmonary disease, including chronic obstructive airway disease (COAD), effusions or cancerous lesions may change the timing of surgery. If tumours or other mediastinal masses are identified, they should be investigated before cardiac procedures are performed.

Cardiac size in adults is determined by assessing the cardiothoracic ratio. The cardiac diameter is normally 50% or less of the thoracic diameter. A ratio greater than 50% indicates cardiac enlargement. Films may also show the presence of calcium in the cardiac valves, coronary arteries and aorta.

The most recent, as well as the previously taken, chest radiographs should be available at the time of surgery. For patients who have required previous sternal operations, the lateral radiograph demonstrates the chest wires, the proximity of the heart to the sternum and the possible extent of pericardial adhesions. Rib notching may be evident on the left side of the thorax because of the tortuous path of hypertrophic intercostal arteries in patients with coarctation of aorta.

Echocardiography and Doppler ultrasonography

Being non-invasive and not requiring the use of ionising radiation, echocardiography is ideal for the evaluation of seriously ill adults. Echocardiography is an integral part of cardiological diagnosis. Cross-sectional images are construed by sweeping the ultrasonic beam across a two-dimensional slice of the heart. Echocardiography should be carried out in all patients in whom a new diagnosis of heart failure is made. It can be used to identify any occult, but treatable, primary cause of heart failure.

Transoesophageal echocardiography (TOE) uses miniaturised trans-ducers incorporated into adapted endoscopes. This allows the heart and great vessels to be studied from within the gastric fundus. It is used to evaluate the cardiac valves and to assess the need to repair versus replace-ment of a valve at operation. Intraoperative TOE is used to test repairs of congenital defects as well as regurgitant valves, and to assess ventricular function.

Echocardiograms from moving blood (Doppler techniques) are advantageous when studying the blood flow within the heart and great vessels.

Main applications

Diagnosis of chest pain

When new ischaemia occurs, the contractile function of the myocardium becomes impaired before the ECG becomes abnormal and before the patient develops symptoms. New abnormalities of wall motion are sensi-tive indicators of ischaemia or developing infarction.

Complications of myocardial infarction

It is invaluable for the prompt diagnosis of the cause relating to sudden haemodynamic collapse in a patient with acute MI. It distinguishes cardiogenic shock from severe left ventricular damage, right ventricular infarction and cardiac rupture with tamponade. It is the best technique for differentiating between acute mitral regurgitation and ventricular septal rupture.

Valvular disease is diagnosed with great accuracy. Obstruction and regurgitation are detected, and their consequences on ventricular dimensions and function are observed. In most patients with valvular heart disease, cardiac catheterisation is required only for coronary arteriography to identify coronary arteries that may be demonstrating significant ischaemia.

Dynamic electrocardiography (Holter monitoring)

From its initiation as a research tool in the 1970s (Campbell, 1993), dynamic electrocardiography or Holter monitoring has developed from a fragile research tool to become a standard and widely available cardiac investigation. It is used for:

- diagnosis of arrhythmias
- assessment of antiarrhythmic drugs
- assessment of pacemaker or implanted cardioverter defibrillator (ICD) function
- detection of ischaemia
- monitoring of blood pressure
- determination of prognosis.

Coronary angiography

Coronary angiography (cardiac catheterisation) is a diagnostic test performed by a cardiologist within the operating room environment of a cardiac catheterisation laboratory; it was developed in 1959. It is the ultimate cardiology test, because it allows the cardiologist to observe the following:

- the left and right coronary arteries for any blockages or narrowings
- the function of the heart valves
- the left ventricle for contractility
- pressures within the heart – normal pressures shown in Table 2.5
- cardiac rate and rhythm.

The following may be indications for performing a cardiac catheterisation:

- increasing shortness of breath
- unstable angina

Table 2.5 Normal cardiovascular pressures

Chamber		Mean (mmHg)	Range (mmHg)
Right atrium	Mean	4	0–8
Right ventricle	Systolic	25	15–30
	End-diastolic	4	0–8
Pulmonary artery	Systolic	25	15–30
	Diastolic	10	5–15
	Mean	15	10–20
Pulmonary artery wedge	Mean	10	5–14
Left atrium	Mean	7	4–12
Left ventricle	Systolic	120	90–140
	End-diastolic	7	4–12
Aorta	Systolic	120	90–140
	Diastolic	70	60–90
	Mean	85	70–105

- ischaemic heart disease
- coronary artery spasm
- after a myocardial infarction
- after open heart surgery
- congenital abnormalities of the heart based on family history
- suspected stenosis of the heart valves
- cardiomyopathy
- transplant assessment
- ventricular septal defect (VSD) before emergency surgery
- cardiac biopsy.

Cardiac catheterisation is usually performed via the femoral artery, but increasingly it is performed using the brachial or radial artery. The procedure takes about 30 minutes on a day-case admission, but a lengthened procedure is required if previously grafted arteries are to be investigated. A provisional diagnosis may be provided on the day of the test, and a number of options may be available, including remaining on the same treatment, increasing medication, proceeding to angioplasty or referral for cardiac surgery. Surgery will not be considered in the absence of any open major artery larger than 1 mm in diameter beyond the obstructing lesion, and in the complete absence of viable myocardium in the area supplied by the stenosed or obstructed arteries.

Patient preparation

Preoperative assessment is performed within a specified period before surgery to ensure that each patient arrives in the operating room in the optimal condition to cope with the physiological changes and stressors associated with surgery, and that patients are less likely to develop perioperative complications. Such assessment should ideally be carried out by an anaesthetist, but nurses are now very involved in this process. It can be argued that a global assessment by another health professional is of limited value because interaction of surgery and anaesthesia with the patient's pre-existing illness is not within their field of expertise. However, nurses provide a holistic assessment that looks at postoperative needs rather than just immediate concerns. The preoperative assessment should not involve a lengthy preoperative stay: the shorter the preoperative stay the less likely the patient is to develop a hospital-acquired infection. After screening for the initial diagnosis or at the assessment before admission for surgery, the value of impending surgery may be deemed minimal, (e.g. coexisting severe non-cardiac conditions with a poor prognosis, such as extreme debility, mental and emotional deterioration and multiple system disease) and may contraindicate bypass grafts.

In an effort to evaluate the preoperative morbidity, classification systems have evolved, the most common being the American Society of Anaesthesiologists' (ASA) Physical Status Classification (Table 2.6). This simple system assigns a number to different degrees of morbidity and it correlates with pre- and postoperative mortality.

Table 2.6 American Society of Anesthesiologists' (ASA) physical status classification

I	Normal, healthy patient
II	Patient with mild systemic disease
III	Patient with systemic disease that limits activity but is not incapacitating
IV	Patient with an incapacitating systemic disease that is a threat to life
V	Moribund patient not expected to survive 24 hours even with an operation

Cardiac surgery continues to be a difficult area for outcome prediction (Turner et al., 1995), but much effort has gone into predicting operative risk based on general preoperative condition and perioperative risk. Two widely used, simple and fairly reliable systems are the Parsonnet Score (Table 2.7) and the EuroScore (European System for Cardiac Operative Risk – Table 2.8). By adding the number allocated to the factor, the risk of mortality can be calculated. The Parsonnet Score was

Table 2.7 The Parsonnet Scoring System

Additive score	Operative mortality (%)
0–4	1 (low risk)
5–9	5 (elevated risk)
10–14	9 (significantly elevated risk)
15–19	17 (high risk)
19+	31 (very high risk)

Patient-related factor	Definition	Score
Sex	Female	1
Morbid obesity	Body mass index > 35	3
Diabetes	Any history of diabetes regardless of duration or treatment. Latent diabetes of pregnancy excluded	3
Hypertension	A history of blood pressure greater than 140/90 mmHg on two occasions, or lower if on medication	3
LV dysfunction	Good (> 50%)	0
	Fair (30–49%) or	2
	Poor (<30%) if known	4
Age	70–74	7
	75–79	12
	>80	20
Reoperation	Second operation	5
	Third (or more)	10
Intra-aortic balloon pump	Before surgery. Do NOT include IABPs inserted prophylactically just before surgery because these represent postoperative support	2
LV aneurysm	Aneurysmectomy	5
Recently failed intervention	No	
	Within 24 h of operation	10
	>24 h, operation on same admission	5
Renal	Dialysis dependency	10
Catastrophic states	For example, acute structural defect, cardiogenic shock, acute renal failure	10–50
Other rare circumstances	For example, paraplegia, pacemaker dependency, congenital heart disease in adults, severe asthma	2–10

Valve surgery-related factors

Mitral valve surgery	Systolic PA pressure < 60 mmHg	5
	Systolic PA pressure ≥ 60 mmHg	8
Aortic valve surgery	AV pressure gradient ≤ 120 mmHg	5
	AV pressure gradient > 120 mmHg	7

Other surgery-related factors

CABG at the time of valve surgery		2

AV, atrioventricular; CABG, coronary artery bypass graft; IABP, intra-aortic balloon pump; LV, left ventricular; PA, pulmonary artery.

Table 2.8 The EuroScore*

Patient-related factors	Definition	Score
Age	Per 5 years or part thereof over 60	1
Sex	Female	1
Chronic pulmonary disease	Long-term use of bronchodilators or steroids for lung disease	1
Extracardiac arteriopathy	Any one or more of the following: claudication, carotid occlusion or > 50% stenosis, previous or planned surgery on the abdominal aorta, limb arteries or carotids	2
Neurological dysfunction	Disease severely affecting ambulation or day-to-day functioning	2
Previous cardiac surgery	Previous surgery requiring opening of the pericardium	3
Serum creatinine	> 200 mmol/l preoperatively	2
Active endocarditis	Patient still under antibiotic treatment for endocarditis at the time of surgery	3
Critical preoperative state	Ventilation before arrival in the anaesthetic room, preoperative inotropic support, intra-aortic balloon counterpulsation (IABP) or preoperative acute renal failure (anuria or oliguria < 10 ml/h)	3
Cardiac-related factors		
Unstable angina	Angina requiring intravenous nitrates until arrival in the operating room	2
LV dysfunction	Moderate (EF 30–50%)	1
	Poor < 30%	3
Recent myocardial infarct	< 90 days	2
Pulmonary hypertension	Systolic PA pressure 60 mmHg	2
Operation-related factors		
Emergency	Carried out on referral before the beginning of the next working day	2
Other than isolated CABG	Major cardiac operation other than or in addition to CABG	2
Surgery on thoracic aorta	Ascending, arch or descending aorta	3
Postinfarct septal rupture		4

*EuroScore – European System for Cardiac Operative Risk Evaluation. Score weights add up to an approximate percentage predicted mortality.
CABG, coronary artery bypass graft; EF, ejection fraction; IABP, intra-aortic balloon pump; LV, left ventricular; PA, pulmonary artery.

the first simple, validated, additive scoring system for predicting risk in cardiac surgery. It is widely used in the UK, but its weakness is that it allows subjective scoring with some variables (e.g. other rare circumstances). The EuroScore is a weighted, additive score similar in concept to the North American Parsonnet Score but based on a European sample of cardiac surgical patients; it represents a considerable improvement on the Parsonnet Score. Both scores concentrate on the mortality risk. The EuroScore does not include diabetes. This is because, although diabetes is recognised as a factor in morbidity, it does not greatly influence the risk of mortality.

Assessment of risk is now important on two counts. The mortality rates of surgeons are under scrutiny from outside sources, and patients are more questioning of health care and should be allowed to make informed decisions on facts. When consent is gained, the degree of risk in relation to mortality and the complications in respect of stroke and renal failure should also be given.

Assessment of risks

Assessment of respiratory risk

In diagnosing heart disease, the degree of dyspnoea experienced is measured, whereas in the preoperative assessment suitability for surgery and risk of complications are assessed. The greatest cause of perioperative morbidity is pulmonary complications and preoperative assessment is aimed at identifying those at risk and decreasing the risk as far as possible. Underlying respiratory disease, smoking and obesity have all been shown to be important. Patients should have already been encouraged to stop smoking when the initial cardiac disorder was diagnosed, but cessation of smoking at least 30 days before surgery reduces the risk of both respiratory and wound infections.

The presence of a recent-onset upper respiratory tract infection is associated with increased airway reactivity, mucous plugging, atelectasis, bronchospasm and pneumonia. Patients who have had a recent infection (within 3–4 weeks preceding surgery) but are asymptomatic pose the greatest risk. All patients with known chronic chest problems should be questioned about the severity of symptoms, whether they have had a recent chest infection and current medication. Pulmonary function tests (PFTs) should be carried out on patients with a chronic disease. These include FEV_1: FVC ratio (ratio of forced expiratory volume in 1 s : forced vital capacity) and peak expiratory flow rate, in addition to arterial blood gases. PFTs are valuable in identifying respiratory diseases, which may be improved preoperatively. Severe reduction in FEV_1/FVC is associated with the need for prolonged intubation; this necessitates a longer stay in intensive care and may expose the patient to increased pulmonary complications. Patients with COAD, including those with asthma, generally have more complications than patients with restrictive conditions, e.g. kyphoscoliosis. If it appears that asthma or COAD could be improved preoperatively, this could necessitate a longer preoperative stay for physiotherapy or systemic steroids.

Evidence of severe pulmonary dysfunction does not contraindicate surgery because it may reflect reversible changes associated with cardiac disease, and it is therefore difficult to define a value below which surgical risk is prohibitive. However, generally an elevated PCO_2 (partial pressure of carbon dioxide) has been identified as a marker of postoperative pulmonary morbidity and mortality.

Assessment of renal disease

A history of renal disease requires close attention to blood urea and electrolyte estimations. Any significant abnormality, such as high or low sodium and potassium values, pH abnormalities or a high creatinine, should be corrected to decrease the risk of interactions with anaesthesia and surgery, which can result in dysrhythmias, cardiac arrest, fits or cerebral depression. An opinion about management from a renal physician may be invaluable in the preparation of patients for surgery. On occasions 24-hour urine collection for urea and creatinine clearance may be requested.

Assessment of diabetes

A diabetic assessment should be carried out before surgery, because people with diabetes undergoing surgery are always a high-risk group. This assessment should involve reviewing current anti-diabetic treatments, previous glycaemic control, known relevant diabetic complications and whether problems have arisen during previous operations. It is important that the patients have good metabolic control, from before induction of anaesthesia until they have recovered completely from the operation. Insulin sensitivity and requirements are altered by the metabolic response to surgery. Operations should not be cancelled on the basis of one random elevated blood glucose, if glycaemic control is normally satisfactory. Where possible, an operation involving patients with diabetes, especially those with type 1 diabetes (insulin-dependent diabetes mellitus), should be the first procedure on the morning operation list. This helps to shorten the preoperative fast for these patients.

Assessment of neurological risk

As a result of the risk of neurological injury caused by of disruption of aortic plaque, preoperative screening of the carotid arteries is sometimes invaluable. Such screening could reduce the prevalence of postoperative stroke. Screening may indicate patients with carotid artery disease who should be monitored for the development of cerebrovascular accident (CVA). Stenosis of the internal carotid artery is often found in asymptomatic patients (Wareing et al., 1992). The potential for a CVA after cardiac surgery increases to 9.9% in the presence of proven stenosis (> 75%) of the carotid artery (Borioni et al., 1994). Detection of a carotid bruit should prompt examination with duplex sonography. If severe (> 70%) stenosis of the carotid artery is detected, clinical judgement is required in relation to the need for carotid endarterectomy and debate continues over the timing of this (Mills, 1995). Endarterectomy is superior to medical treatment for these patients. Medical therapy includes oral daily doses of anticoagulants. The risk of perioperative stroke is also increased in patients with atrial rhythm disorders, left ventricular thrombi and severe aortic atheroma.

Patients requiring cardiac surgery as a result of coronary atherosclerosis will also invariably demonstrate atherosclerotic changes elsewhere. This may be most notable in the legs and, therefore, patients should be assessed for peripheral vascular disease that can be superficially achieved by assessing the presence of femoral, post-popliteal and post-tibial pulses. Absence of these pulses by palpitation may prompt a Doppler test, but it does not necessarily denote a contraindication for surgery. However, the use of the saphenous vein for bypass grafts in these patients may result in delayed healing. It is also relevant in the postoperative period for all patients, particularly those requiring intra-aortic balloon counterpulsation or anti-embolism stockings, both of which are contraindicated in the presence of peripheral vascular disease.

If the patient requires coronary artery bypass grafts, the legs should be assessed for varicose veins or previous surgery. Their presence may prevent the use of the saphenous vein from the affected limb(s). The suitability of the radial and ulnar artery as a conduit should be assessed by Allen's test. Any delay in the resolution of the blanching could prevent the use of the radial artery. Further investigation by Doppler ultrasonography will provide a more accurate report on the patency of vessels.

A patient with a history of alcoholism or alcohol abuse has an increased risk of intraoperative bleeding, in addition to postoperative hepatic dysfunction or delirium. It may also affect the type of surgery performed and subsequent treatment (e.g. the use of a metal or tissue valve prosthesis).

Preoperative blood tests

Bloods need to be taken for routine screening and a crossmatch. The collection of blood samples is an underestimated skill. The value of subsequent laboratory tests is dependent on the sample being taken from the patient correctly. One of the errors commonly seen is a haemolysed sample, which can give falsely high records of potassium and magnesium. Integrated blood collection systems have far less scope to spoil samples than those involving separate needle syringe and bottles. When using a separate syringe and bottle, the largest bore needle possible should be used (usually a 21 gauge). The plunger should be drawn slowly back, and the needle must be removed before the blood is expelled into the containers. Small-bore needles increase the chances of haemolysis occurring, particularly if the sample is drawn quickly. Table 2.9 shows the normal ranges for blood results.

Table 2.9 Normal blood values

Sodium	135–145 mmol/l
Potassium	3.6–5.0 mmol/l
Creatinine	60–125 µmol/l
Urea	2.5–7.1 mmol/l
Glucose	3.5–9.0 mmol/l
Creatine kinase	15–185 µl
Asparate transaminase	13–45 µl
Albumin	35–50 g/l
Calcium	2.10–2.60 mmol/l
Alkaline phosphatase	30–100 µl
Total bilirubin	0–17 mmol/l
Cholesterol	3.0–5.2 mmol/l
Haemoglobin	
• Men	14–18 g/dl (= g/100 ml)
• Women	12–16 g/dl (= g/100 ml)
White blood cells	$4-11 \times 10^9/l$
Platelets	$150-500 \times 10^9/l$

A full blood count is required, including the international normalised ratio (INR), the activated partial thromboplastin time (APPT), and the platelet count. If any abnormality is detected, this should be addressed before surgery. Electrolyte, urea, creatinine and glucose levels should ideally be within normal limits, but an elevated creatinine may require investigation and treatment before surgery. Liver function tests (LFTs), including bilirubin, alkaline phosphatase, alanine transaminase (ALT), asparate transaminase (AST), albumin and serum amylase, are all useful markers. Elevated levels may be suggestive of hepatitis or cirrhosis and may warrant investigation before surgery.

Although the indications for blood transfusion may have been modified as a result of blood-borne disease, blood transfusions can be a life-saving measure for patients with reduced oxygen-carrying capacity, coagulopathies or hypovolaemia. Blood availability is very necessary and at least 4 units of packed red blood cells are generally ordered for cardiac surgical patients. This blood should be in the operating room for the start of surgery.

Skin cleansing and shaving

To reduce the incidence of wound infections, a recognised complication of any surgery (see Chapter 9), attention is required to skin hygiene and shaving. Hibiscrub showers are advocated before cardiac surgery to prevent wound contamination by organisms on the skin. The recent and continuing escalation in the incidence of methicillin-resistant *Staphylococcus aureus* (MRSA) has caused some hospitals to promote a 5-day course of Hibiscrub showers, including the hair. Patients unable to shower are bed bathed. Patients previously identified as MRSA positive should receive a 5-day course of Hibiscrub showers in addition to Bactrodan or Naseptin nasal cream.

The shaving of operative sites started at the beginning of the twentieth century and is the subject of ongoing debate. In the past, cardiac patients often had full body shaves, but this practice has fortunately been abandoned. Practicality suggests that hair must be removed when it might interfere with the incision, or when it would compromise placement of postoperative dressings. A heavy growth of hair could impede the placement of grounding pads and sterile adhesive drapes. Most male patients do have hair removed along the sternal midline, from the sternal notch to just above the umbilicus, but female patients rarely require hair removal. In coronary artery bypass patients, the skin along the inner aspect of the leg (in the path of the greater saphenous vein) may be shaved. The forearm may be shaved to prevent discomfort on removal of plaster securing intravenous access lines. Surgical wound infections continue to be a serious complication of surgery. The method of hair removal can be a factor in reducing infection rates. It is thought that abandoning shaving in favour of clipping could result in a reduced incidence of infections. The literature promotes caution with regard to shaving operation sites. Most research advocates shaving with disposable razors as close to the operating room as possible, namely in the operating suite itself. However, shaving at this time can still cause superficial cuts. Disposable clippers are now available, which can shave hair effectively, but are less likely to cut the skin.

Discontinuation of medication

The *Drugs and Therapeutics Bulletin* offered suggestions about the stopping of medication before surgery (Collier, 1999). Cardiac drugs, such as anti-hypertensives, anti-angina and anti-arrhythmia medications, should be continued up to surgery. This may prevent rebound hypertension and recurrence of ischaemia, and provides for a more stable anaesthetic. Diuretics of a potassium-sparing nature should be omitted on the morning of surgery, but thiazides or loop diuretics should not be withdrawn. Digoxin should be withheld unless it is required to control ventricular rate. An increased sensitivity to digoxin can occur in the early postoperative period as a result of fluid and electrolyte shifts during surgery (Harlan et al., 1995).

Warfarin is usually withdrawn from about 4 days preoperatively to allow the INR to fall below 1.5, a level considered safe for surgery to be performed (White et al., 1995) and, if necessary, heparin can be substituted until surgery. When there is too little time to withdraw warfarin, fresh frozen plasma (10–15 ml/kg) is given (Travis et al., 1989). Aspirin may be continued for patients undergoing cardiac surgery, although it appears to be customarily stopped for 7 days before surgery to allow for adequate platelet function. Although there is increased risk of perioperative bleeding if aspirin is not discontinued, there is evidence that, if it is discontinued, ischaemic events could occur before surgery, and there may be reduced graft patency postoperatively (Matsuzaki et al., 1999). Other non-steroidal anti-inflammatory drugs should be stopped for a similar time to allow for platelet function.

For patients taking oral contraceptives and hormone replacement therapy, these should be discontinued several weeks before major surgery to lower the risk of venous thrombosis.

Patients usually have a premedication in the form of a sedative, and this may be prescribed as a night sedative on the evening before surgery, with a similar dose up to 2 hours before surgery. The premedication may include continuous oxygen therapy, but this appears to depend on consultant preference rather than evidence-based practice.

Consent

With the increase in liability, the gaining of consent is much more focused. The days when patients were merely passive participants in health care are gone, and all patients now require the full nature of the surgery, and its connected risks, to be explained. In addition to preventing a breakdown in communication, consent should be gained by a person capable of performing the surgery. Once a consent form is signed it remains valid for a period of 3 months. If a delay in surgery occurs, despite the validity of the consent form, it is important to ensure that, first, the patient still requires surgery and, second, the physical condition of the patient has not altered. Any alteration, which may ultimately change the risk of surgery, should require consent being re-sought, the risks having been explained to the patient.

When the operation is being explained to the patient, the patient should have the opportunity to refuse treatment, or certain therapies associated with the operation. This may be of particular relevance to certain religious groups such as Jehovah's Witnesses, who usually do not allow blood transfusions. For these patients, the risk of haemorrhage should be discussed and alternative treatments considered such as auto-transfusion.

Information needs to be given to the patient, but not only for the purposes of consent. It has been recognised for several decades that preoperative information can have a positive effect on patients postoperatively. It can, in particular, reduce the patient's experience of pain and anxiety. It is important that the patient and relatives know what to expect with regard to invasive lines, environment and normal procedures.

The waiting period for surgery is thought to be a most stressful time for patients and their relatives. During this time, the main needs of the family are having control of the situation, privacy, being able to express emotions, information, and access to the surgeon in order that he or she can answer questions. The main information needs are concerning the operation, e.g. date and time, how long the patient is going to be in intensive care, when he or she can go home afterwards, when he or she can resume exercise and when he or she can return to work.

Fasting

Before the elective administration of anaesthesia, it is customary practice to fast patients for a minimum of 4 hours. This has the intention of allowing the stomach to empty, to reduce the incidence of perioperative or postoperative vomiting and regurgitation, and the possible risk of aspiration into the lungs, which may result in respiratory complications. However, this theoretical 4- to 6-hour preoperative fasting appears to result in periods of abstinence that might be better termed 'preoperative starvation'. Preoperative starvation could lead to a state of catabolism, which may be detrimental to the patient undergoing major surgery (Torrence, 1991); 4–6 hours is sufficient to account for the variable time required for gastric emptying of solids, but clear fluids are appropriate for up to 2 hours preoperatively (Chapman, 1996).

Much of the preoperative preparation is for the postoperative period. The spouse needs to anticipate the recovery process in order to reduce distress associated with unexpected events, e.g. pain, depression. The spouse should be encouraged to visit the intensive care/recovery area, where there is the opportunity to see other patients recovering from cardiac surgery, and to see equipment. It is important to inform them that patients do not remember experiences in the intensive care/recovery area, and that their behaviour during the initial stages of their recovery may be foreign to their normal behaviour. This may reduce the distress of seeing a family member who appears to be out of touch with reality.

The wait on the surgeon's list is the prime time to facilitate the complete recovery from surgery by promoting a healthy lifestyle. Cessation of cigarette smoking is a primary objective in the preoperative and postoperative period. The preadmission period on the waiting list is an especially good time to carry out patient teaching because there may be less stress at this time compared with the immediate preoperative period. The optimum time before admission to provide information is 14 days, and many centres have now established preadmission clinics to facilitate this teaching.

Cancellations

Most patients become understandably anxious when they are initially referred for cardiac surgery and, therefore, a person who is admitted to hospital to undergo surgery often passes through an extremely stressful period before surgery is performed. Patients are psychologically and physically prepared for cardiac surgery and, on most occasions, if a patient's operation is cancelled, this occurs on the day of the operation, usually within hours of the patient going to the anaesthetic room. Not all patients receive warning that cancellation may occur and, on isolated occasions, a patient may have been taken to the anaesthetic room, only to have the operation cancelled as the result of an unforeseen emergency. In these cases, the premedication is already taking effect so the patient may be unaware that the operation has been cancelled for many hours. It is the medical staff who usually explain the cancellation to the patient.

Rescheduling of operations differs between centres. Patients may remain as inpatients and take the next available slot, whereas others go home to be readmitted at a prearranged date. Allowing the patient to remain a patient avoids the trauma of patients going home feeling anxious and frightened.

References

Borioni R, Garofalo M, Pellegrino A, Actis Dato G, Chiarello L (1994) Stroke prevention and carotid artery disease in cardiac surgical patients. *Ann Thorac Surg* **58**: 1788–9.

Campbell R (1993) Dynamic electrocardiography (Holter monitoring). *Med Int* 338–45.

Chapman A (1996) Current theory and practice in a study of preoperative fasting. *Nursing Standard* **10**(8): 33–6.

Collier J (1999) Drugs in the peri-operative period 1. Stopping or continuing drugs around surgery. *Drugs Ther Bull* **37**(8): 59–64.

Dargie HJ (1993) Exercise electrocardiography. *Med Int* 346–50.

Harlen BJ, Starr A, Harwin FM (1995) *Illustrated Handbook of Cardiac Surgery*. New York: Springer.

Matsuzaki K, Matsui K, Haraguchi N, Nagan I, Okabe H, Asou T (1999) Ischaemic heart attacks following cessation of aspirin before coronary artery bypass surgery – a report of two cases. *Ann Thorac Cardiovasc Surg* **5**: 121–2.

Mills S (1995) Risk factors for cerebral injury and cardiac surgery. *Ann Thorac Surg* **59**: 1356–8.

Torrence C (1991) Preoperative nutrition, fasting and the surgical patient. *Surg Nurse* **4**(4): 4–8.

Turner JS, Morgan CJ, Thakrar B, Pepper JR (1995) Difficulties in predicting outcome in cardiac surgery patients. *Crit Care Med* **23**: 1843–50.

Travis S, Wray R, Harrison K (1989) Perioperative anticoagulation control. *Br J Surg* **76**: 1107–8.

Wareing TH, Davila-Roman VG, Barzilai B, Murphy SE, Kouchoukos NT (1992) Management of the severely atherosclerotic ascending aorta during cardiac operations: a strategy for detection and treatment. *J Thorac Cardiovasc Surg* **103**: 453–62.

White RH, McKittrick T, Hutchinson R, Twitchell J (1995) Temporary discontinuation of Warfarin therapy: changes in the international normalised ratio. *Ann Intern Med* 122: 40–2.

Further reading

Dripps RD et al. (1961) Role of anaesthesia in surgical mortality. *JAMA* **178**: 261.

Fraser A (1993) Echocardiography and Doppler ultrasound. *Med Int* 330–7.

Shaw D (1993) Palpitation and syncope. *Med Int* 285–7.

CHAPTER 3

Intraoperative care

Induction of anaesthesia

The period immediately after entry into the operating room and that during the placement of venous and arterial lines can be stressful to the patient, resulting in increased heart rate and blood pressure. Non-invasive monitoring of blood pressure, ECG and pulse oximetry are started immediately.

The basic anaesthesia principles of avoidance of hypotension and hypoxia are followed because myocardial oxygenation is critical. Myocardial necrosis and ventricular arrhythmias can occur during induction of anaesthesia as a result of an abnormal myocardial oxygen supply:demand ratio, caused either by a fall in oxygen supply secondary to hypotension or hypoxia, or by an increase in myocardial oxygen demand that cannot be met by an increase in oxygen supply. Myocardial oxygen demand may increase during the period of induction, particularly during intubation, and patients with coronary disease seem to be more prone to this increase.

Oral intubation occurs after induction of anaesthesia, and the patient has been oxygenated for at least 1 minute. The size of the endotracheal tube selected will depend on the individual, but for most female patients a size of 7.5–8.5 i.d. (internal diameter) is used, and in male patients 8.5–9.5 i.d.

Other lines are also placed in the anaesthetic room: a central venous pressure line to monitor filling pressures; a radial arterial line; a urinary catheter; a peripheral intravenous access line for the administration of medication; and, in some centres, a sheath to facilitate pulmonary artery catheter placement. Before the siting of an arterial line, an Allen's test is performed to determine the adequacy of collateral (ulnar artery) blood flow to the hand. The radial artery is cannulated to facilitate continuous blood pressure monitoring and to provide access for arterial blood sampling.

Surgical preparation of the patient

Antimicrobial agents are applied to the skin as expeditiously as possible in the form of iodine or chlorhexidine. Iodine provides for antimicrobial activity for 8 hours compared with the 4 hours provided by chlorhexidine gluconate, although it may cause an allergic reaction in some patients. Skin preparation of the groin is recommended for all cardiac surgical patients, because access to femoral arteries may be required for cannulation, intra-aortic balloon or pressure monitoring line insertion. If the saphenous vein is to be removed, a circumferential leg preparation (up to and including the feet) is recommended.

Draping

Special consideration is given to bypass lines and multiple surgical sites that may be required. The following are the goals for draping:

- exposure of the surgical sites
- maintenance of sterility of the field, including instruments, equipment and bypass lines
- ensuring bypass lines and other items passed off the field are securely attached to drapes
- ensuring that required tubes and cables are easily and quickly accessible.

The supine position is the most commonly used position for cardiac surgery because it exposes the whole anterior chest, both groins for femoral access and, when needed, legs for saphenous vein harvest. A left full lateral or semilateral position is used for operations requiring access to the descending thoracic aorta. Right lateral positions may be used for repeat mitral valve procedures.

Most cardiac procedures are performed by a median sternotomy. This incision provides the best overall access to the heart chambers, results in the least respiratory impairment and the least discomfort for the patient, and an optimum exposure for the institution of cardiopulmonary bypass (CPB). It is the incision of choice for pericardectomy, thymectomy and anterior mediastinal tumours. The skin incision is made in the midline, from below the sternal notch to the linea alba below the xiphoid process. The sternum is split using an air-driven saw. The skin incision and the sternotomy (the exposure of the heart) may stimulate an increase in heart rate and blood pressure, which will require treatment either by increasing the depth of the anaesthesia or by the use of vasoactive agents

Repeat sternotomy is becoming more frequent, especially in patients who have undergone coronary artery bypass grafts (CABGs), but whose progressive coronary atherosclerosis and vein graft disease have caused recurring angina. The operation is technically more demanding because of dense adhesions that form between the pericardium, the great vessels, the retrosternum and bypass conduits, which makes sternotomy and dissection of the heart more hazardous and identification of vessels more difficult. These are all reflected in a higher morbidity and mortality rate.

A new technique for CABGs, a single left internal mammary artery to the left anterior descending artery, using a left anterior small thoracotomy (LAST), has now been developed but not all patients are eligible for this technique. The procedure enables surgery to be performed without the use of CPB or cardioplegia. A 5cm anterior thoracotomy incision is used in preference to a median sternotomy. LAST can be performed on the left anterior descending artery as long as the artery is not calcified or its location is not substernal or intramyocardial, when a traditional median sternotomy will be used.

Cardiopulmonary bypass

The first successful use of mechanically supported circulation and respiration during open heart surgery was performed by Gibbon in 1953 (after 23 years of research), on a woman with a septal defect; his work was a major contribution to the development of modern CPB (Seifert, 1994). It is almost exclusive to heart surgery and has important physiological and biochemical effects that may influence the postoperative care needs of the patient. Hypothermia, non-pulsatile perfusion and hormone release all commonly occur, and these and haemodilution may cause a substantial increase in plasma noradrenaline and adrenaline levels.

Venous blood is drained from the right side of the heart via the superior vena cava and the inferior vena cava, arterialised in the oxygenator and pumped back into the aorta. To prevent thrombosis within the bypass circuit from exposure of the blood to a foreign surface, the patient's system is anticoagulated with heparin. Heparin prolongs whole blood clotting time, thrombin time, partial thromboplastin time and prothrombin time, and usually has a platelet-inhibiting effect. It is given before cannulation for CPB or before clamping of the blood vessels. Heparin may be given by the surgeon directly into the right atrium or by the anaesthetist through the central line. Administration peripherally is avoided to ensure that the heparin reaches the central circulation.

To determine whether adequate heparinisation has been achieved, the activated clotting time (ACT) is measured about 3 min after the heparin is given. During the bypass, periodic ACTs are measured, and additional heparin is administered to maintain the ACT well above 400 seconds (three times above normal.). If patients have been on long-term heparin therapy before surgery (e.g. unstable angina), they may demonstrate heparin resistance. The reason for this is unclear but the situation is usually resolved by increasing the amount of heparin.

Protamine sulphate, despite its own anticoagulating properties, is given to reverse the effects of heparin. A calculated dosage of 1–1.3 times the total heparin dose is normally administered, and the ACT results can guide additional protamine infusions. Protamine infusion is associated with systemic hypotension and decreased systemic vascular resistance and, in some cases, a full anaphylactic reaction may occur. In some units, the infusion is commenced before removal of the arterial cannula so that volume may be given to maintain an adequate blood pressure or CPB can be rapidly restored if any adverse effects are encountered.

The patient's height and weight are used to calculate body surface area. Standard bypass usually maintains flows between 1.8 l/min per m^2 (low flow) and 2.4 l/min per m^2 (high flow), moderate systemic temperature of 26°C and 30°C, and moderate haemodilution with the haematocrit between 20% and 30%. The flow can be pulsatile. High flow is usually maintained at normothermia and during cooling, and re-warming. Low flow is satisfactory during hypothermia because body oxygen consumption at 30°C is half that at 37°C. Low flow decreases bronchial flow and non-coronary collateral flow, and can facilitate an operation.

Adverse effects of CPB

Patients tend to have some physiological systemic inflammatory response to bypass. This is evidenced by prolonged pulmonary insufficiency, excessive accumulation of extravascular water, elevated temperature, vasoconstriction, coagulopathy, and varying degrees of renal or other organ dysfunction. The main reason for the physiological response is the exposure of blood to the abnormal surfaces of the CPB circuit, the presence of hypothermia, altered blood flow and damage caused by the roller pump, all of which initiate a systemic inflammatory response.

During bypass, platelets are depleted in numbers and activity. Their granules become depleted and some of their contents can be demonstrated in circulating blood. Individual clotting factors are reduced in concentration because of consumption as a result of exposing blood to foreign surfaces despite heparinisation.

Hypothermia

Hypothermia is used to decrease metabolic rate and reduce damage caused by ischaemia during surgery, thereby preserving function. It has several uses:

- decreases metabolic rate
- decreases tissue oxygen demands
- protects the brain
- reduces the risk of ischaemic tissue damage to the heart, protecting other vital organs from hypoxia.

Cooling to 15°C in the presence of oxygen reduces oxygen consumption to a fifth of the rate at normal body temperature. Myocardial protection is provided by a range of techniques: cold crystalloid cardioplegia; cold blood cardioplegia; and, more recently, intermittent warm blood cardioplegia.

Core warming is initiated before discontinuation of CPB, and most patients are normothermic at the time of terminating CPB. Spontaneous ventricular contractions usually occur at temperatures of 30–32°C and, if necessary, a fibrillating heart can be defibrillated at 33°C.

The heart is irritable, and may fibrillate if inadvertently touched, but this can be reversed by internal defibrillation with specifically designed paddles. The standard level of energy current for internal defibrillation is 10–20 joules (J), and this will be effective in 90% of cases. Lower settings may require repeat shocks and higher settings can cause myocardial necrosis.

The perfusionist's primary function is to provide CPB facilities for cardiac surgeons, with the aim of providing the best perfusion to enable optimal operating conditions and for maintaining adequate perfusion of the tissues while on bypass. The perfusionist is responsible for preparing the extracorporeal circuit for all procedures. The circuit is assembled from disposable components: membrane oxygenator, heater/roller, arterial line filter and tubing. The circuit is primed, commonly with 1 litre Hartmann's solution, 500 ml Gelofusine, 6000 units heparin and 0.5 g/kg body weight of 20% mannitol. This is primarily to ensure that all dead space is filled and air free before initiating CPB.

When CPB has been established, the perfusionist maintains adequate blood flow to the patient while monitoring blood gas and electrolyte status, blood pressure and ACT. As a sedated or anaesthetised patient will not be aware of hypoglycaemia, regular perioperative blood glucose monitoring is undertaken. After surgery, insulin should be given intravenously rather than subcutaneously, and this should be continued until the patient recommences his or her usual diet.

During surgery, and particularly for patients who have refused blood transfusion, a cell saver may be employed. Cell saving has the following advantages:

• No transfusion reactions
• Reduced demand on the blood bank
• Less disease risk to the patient.

It is contraindicated for patients with sepsis or malignancy.

Intraoperative haemostasis should be obtained by meticulous surgical technique in preference to extensive use of blood products. In about 50% of patients undergoing primary coronary artery bypass grafts, and with no preoperative anaemia, no homologous blood should be required. Use of donor bank blood can be minimised in a number of ways: preoperative and intraoperative donation; ultrafiltration device within the pump oxygenator system; reinfusion of shed blood drained from chest tubes (autotransfusion); and collection of intraoperative shed blood, i.e. cell saver. (This 'cell saver' is then washed, the erythrocytes concentrated and the patient's blood collected via the suction unit from the operative field and directed into a sterile reservoir. This blood is centrifuged, removing the platelets, activated clotting factors, operative debris and 99% of the heparin. The discard is collected in a waste bag, the red blood cells washed and returned to the patient via an infusion.)

Cardioplegia

Hypothermia reduces oxygen consumption but metabolic requirements can be lessened further by reducing cardiac muscle activity. The infusion of a cold hyperkalaemic solution provides myocardial cooling and inhibits membrane depolarisation and propagation of the action potential. The resulting cardioplegia produces a reversible diastolic arrest, which allows the surgeon to perform delicate procedures on a quiet operative field. Infusions are needed at intervals of about 20 min because the cardioplegic solution eventually washes out as the myocardium re-warms.

Perfusion of the coronary arteries with cardioplegic solution provides the best preservation of myocardial function during extracorporeal bypass, at a time when the heart is not continuously perfused with blood. The purpose of chemical cardioplegia is to prevent the consequences of ischaemia by providing an environment in which myocardial injury is avoided by meeting reduced energy demands. It should maintain the heart in quiet arrest for as long as necessary to provide the surgeon with an optimum operative field.

Coronary artery bypass grafting without the use of CPB is being developed. If the technique proves to be successful, it offers the potential of a decreased stay in intensive care, earlier hospital discharge and reduced morbidity. The major problem with this technique is that the anaesthetist has to maintain cardiovascular stability during the bypass procedure and the surgeon has to attempt stabilisation of the heart, in order to perform the anastomosis in a safe fashion.

Choice of donor site in coronary artery bypass grafts

A coronary artery bypass graft is the attachment of a conduit directly to the coronary artery, at a point distal to the stenosis (Figure 3.1). Blocked arteries in the limbs have been replaced since the 1950s, but not until 1967 were the coronary arteries tackled when Rene Favaloro, a cardiac surgeon at the Cleveland Clinic, Ohio, inaugurated the coronary artery bypass operation (Hurt, 1996). Initially, reverse segments of autologous saphenous vein were used as conduits. The long saphenous vein is expendable, available in sufficient length, appropriately sized to match the coronary arteries, capable of reaching beyond the stenosis of all diseased arteries and sufficiently pliable to allow easy suturing (Kirklin et al., 1991). When this vein is not available the short saphenous vein may be used.

The harvesting of the saphenous vein is a crucial step. Harvesting time varies depending on the length of vein and the size of the leg (Wolff et al., 1997). Improper handling of the vein and subsequent injury can jeopar-

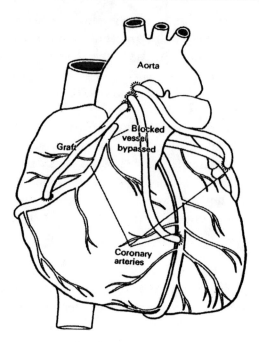

Figure 3.1 Coronary artery bypass grafts. From K Jarrett (1976), *Triumphs of Medicine,* Paul Elek Ltd.

dise the successful outcome of an otherwise properly performed procedure. The vein is irrigated with a balanced salt solution and any additional branches ligated. The vein is removed with very gentle handling and sharp dissection of the vein and its branches. The branches are tied, clipped and divided.

The left internal mammary artery (internal thoracic artery) is now widely used and is the conduit of choice for revascularisation of the left anterior descending (LAD) artery. The internal mammary artery (IMA), left attached at its origin from the left subclavian artery, is mobilised from the chest wall and usually anastomosed to the LAD artery, the harvesting taking about 20 min. The patency of the internal mammary artery graft to the LAD coronary artery is thought to be around 90–95% at 10 years, compared with a saphenous vein graft patency of 40–60% (Dietl et al., 1993). Use of the IMA to the LAD carries an improved 10-year survival, but its use has an increased risk of sternal wound infections, especially in patients with type 1 diabetes. It is thought that arterial grafts may be more resistant to atherosclerotic changes than venous grafts, possibly because arteries are accustomed to high-pressure systems, and tend not to develop accelerated atherosclerosis, in contrast to veins (Spence and Gray, 1994).

The growing incidence of coronary reoperations has increased the need for alternative conduits in situations when the saphenous vein and IMA cannot be used, including patients with previous bilateral vein stripping, and extensive varicosities or the presence of vessels that are too small or too fragile. The following are other conduits (Table 3.1) that have been used: cephalic vein, basilic vein, right gastroepiploic artery, radial artery, splenic artery and inferior epigastric artery. The most commonly used of these are the cephalic and basilic veins, but these appear to carry a higher failure rate. In addition, positioning for access to the vein is cumbersome and difficult. The skin incision may be disfiguring and uncomfortable.

A number of reports have suggested differences in technique required for women in contrast to men. Coronary artery bypass grafts in women appear to be more technically difficult, possibly as a result of anatomical differences. The heart and coronary arteries of women are generally smaller

Table 3.1 The uses and patency of various conduits in coronary artery bypass grafts

Harvested vessel	Uses
Short saphenous vein	Often the vein of choice when the greater saphenous is not present. It has been found to have acceptable patency rates when used for lower extremity revascularisation
Cephalic and basilic veins	Can be used but the patency rates are lower than those achieved by leg veins. Patency rates are suggested as 57% at 2 years and 47% at 4.6 years
Gastroepiploic artery	This was first described as an alternative conduit in 1987. A retrogastric route is preferable for the right coronary and circumflex systems, and an anterogastric route for the left anterior descending. Reports of early graft patency are encouraging at 95% patency between 2 and 4 years. Long-term results are not yet available, but it is suggested to be favourable as a result of similarities to the internal mammary artery (IMA). Technically this artery is more difficult to handle and suture, and is more prone to spasm than the IMA. It may have serious consequences for future abdominal surgery
Inferior epigastric artery	Can be harvested, and results are thought to be favourable, initial reports suggesting 80% patency after 1 year
Radial artery	The use of this artery was first reported in 1973, but it was little used as a result of high occlusion rates of 50–60% in the first year. This has recently received new interest with accompanying diltiazem to prevent spasm, when a patency rate of 93.5% at 9 months is observed. Risks with this route include possible hand ischaemia, graft occlusion, localised infection, dysaesthesia and impaired mobility

than those in men, and this can affect anastomotic techniques. Graft patency is lower in women: smaller vessels, thin-walled saphenous veins, and more diabetes and hypertension have all been suggested as reasons. Another factor may be that women are usually referred for surgery later in the course of the disease, by which time ventricular function is poorer.

Transmyocardial revascularistion involves using a laser beam to create fine holes in the left ventricle to improve myocardial perfusion. It is a therapeutic option for end-stage coronary artery disease if no other revascularisation intervention is suitable. Treatment should be offered after maximum medical therapy is unsuccessful, but should be avoided if the left ejection fraction is less than 40%. Trials into this treatment have now been completed, and overall it is not seen as a good option.

Coronary endarterectomy

This is usually reserved for the removal of plaque from the coronary artery system when it is occluded and no distal branches are available for anastomosis. This technique was refined in 1967 by Sol Sobel, who injected a powerful jet of carbon dioxide gas into an artery by hypodermic syringe. Endarterectomy of the left coronary artery system is performed less often and remains controversial

Valve surgery

In 1948 surgeons would open a diseased mitral valve by inserting a finger into it. Later it was realised that the best answer was to replace failing valves with artificial ones. In 1952, Charles A Hufnagel, an American surgeon, inserted a plastic valve into the descending part of the aorta in the chest to take over from a diseased aortic valve, providing partial haemodynamic relief. Three years later, surgeons started to replace diseased valves in the subcoronary position, with valves taken from human cadavers. Since 1989, there has been a steady increase in the number of valves replaced, particularly among the elderly population (Taylor, 1997). The trend appears to be a preference for mechanical valves over bioprostheses, from single-leaflet to bileaflet mechanical valves, less use of pericardial bioprosthesis and a move towards stentless prosthesis.

Metal versus tissue valves

The first popular model of prosthetic valve is the Starr–Edwards ball valve used in 1960 and designed by the America heart specialist Albert

Starr and aircraft engineer ML Edwards. Since then, various designs and material have been used as substitutes for native cardiac valves, but the ideal replacement has yet to be identified. Valve prostheses are of two types – mechanical and biological – and both have advantages and disadvantages. The current choice is among three widely used types of mechanical prosthesis: ball valve (Starr–Edwards), tilting disc (Medtronic Hall) and bileaflet (Cardiomedics, St Jude Valve), and the porcine xenograft bioprostheses.

The selection of a prosthetic valve is a highly individualised process and is influenced by the presence of cardiac arrhythmias, coexisting coronary artery disease, ventricular function, age and contraindications to anticoagulation (Mylonakis et al., 1999). Mechanical valves appear to be the best choice for patients without coronary artery disease in their 60s and 70s, but they require close monitoring for the development of thrombotic obstruction. The incidence of prosthetic valve thrombosis (i.e. the formation, development or presence of a thrombus) ranges from 0.1% to 5.7% per patient per year, and is highest in mitral valves and in the setting of inadequate anticoagulation therapy (Mylonakis et al., 1999). Early morbidity (30 days) for first-time valve replacement patients has declined from 7.37% in 1986 to 4.44% in 1994, despite the increasing average age. The major factor influencing long-term survival after valve replacement is age. Survival after 19 years for patients younger than 70 at the age of implant is 65% compared with 42% for older patients (Taylor, 1997).

A minimally invasive procedure for performing repair or replacement of the heart valve has recently been developed. This procedure aims to simplify the technique of valve repair and the trauma associated with it. One such procedure is termed 'port access' – minimally invasive valve surgery in which CPB is still used, but sternotomy is not necessary.

Sternal wires

Once the surgeon has achieved haemostasis, stainless steel wire sutures are passed around or through the sternum. Generally five to six are inserted. These wires are permanent and generally do not cause any problems to the patient, although occasional allergic reactions are identified.

Occasionally, delayed sternal closure is necessary in patients whose clotting mechanism is impaired, and this may predispose to a significant risk of bleeding and cardiac tamponade. These patients are returned to intensive care with the sternum left open, but the skin closed. Once the coagulopathy is corrected the patient is returned to the operating room for sternal closure. This is normally within 48 hours.

Creation of a pericardial window

Pericardiotomy via an anterior thoracotomy or subxiphoid approach can be used to drain the pericardium.

Permanent pacemakers

The initial cardiac pacemakers were external, the battery being connected to the heart by a wire running through the vein. These were adequate for hospitalised patients but not for permanent use. The first internal pacemaker was implanted by Dr Ake Sennin from Sweden in 1960. Most pacemakers are now implanted by cardiologists under local anaesthesia, requiring the patient to remain in hospital less than 24 hours.

References

Dietl CA, Madigan NP, Menapace FF et al. (1993) Results of coronary artery bypass grafting using multiple arterial conduits. *J Cardiovasc Surg* **34**: 513–16.
Gibbon JH (1954) Application of mechanical heart and lung apparatus to cardiac surgery. *Minn Med* **37**: 171.
Hurt R (1996) *The History of Cardiothoracic Surgery from Early Times*. Carnforth, Lancashire: Parthenon Publishing Co., p. 33.
Kirklin J, and American College of Cardiology/American Heart Association Task Force on Assessment and Diagnostic and Therapeutic Cardiovascular procedures (1991) The coronary artery bypass operation. *J Am Coll Cardiol* **17**(3): 543–89.
Mylonakis E, Kon D, Moulton A et al. (1999) Thrombosis of mitral valve prosthesis presenting as abdominal pain. *Heart Lung* 28 110–113
Seifert P (1994) *Cardiac Surgery*. St Louis, MO: Mosby, p. 185.
Spence P, Gray LA (1994) New conduits for coronary artery bypass: great promise for improved outcome from coronary artery surgery. *J Ky Med Assoc* **92**: 35–58.
Taylor K (1997) The United Kingdom Heart Valve Registry: The first 10 years. *Heart* **77**: 295–6.
Wolff CA, Scott C, Banks T (1997) The radial artery: An exciting alternative conduit in coronary artery bypass grafting. *Crit Care Nursing* **17**(5): 34–9.

Further reading

Downes R (1997) The role of the cardiac perfusionist. *Br J Theatre Nursing* **7**(3): 18.
Durdey E (1997) Practical cell saving. *Br J Nursing* **7**(3): 16–17.

CHAPTER 4

The respiratory needs of the cardiac surgical patient

The principal goal in the care of patients recovering from general anaesthesia is to protect the airway and ensure adequate oxygenation. The care following cardiac surgery is no exception, except that this is initially achieved with the assistance of an endotracheal tube and a ventilator.

For almost two decades patients were nursed on an intensive care unit immediately after surgery, and were routinely ventilated for periods greater than 8 hours. The purpose of this ventilated period was to ensure complete recovery from anaesthesia, to maintain haemodynamic stability and to allow the patient to rest, which ultimately reduced myocardial oxygen demand. Over the past decade, with continued improvements in cardiac surgery, it has been realised that a routine period of ventilation (i.e. > 6 hours) and the intensive care environment are not required, and could even be detrimental to a patient's recovery. Early extubation has been defined, in relation to cardiac surgery, as extubation of the patient within 8 hours of leaving the cardiac operating room (Higgins, 1992).

The move away from routine ventilation overnight, proposed by Lefemine and Harken (1966), may have been prompted by the increasing waiting lists and the need to speed up a patient's recovery, but it has proved to be of benefit to both the institutions and the patients. During the 1990s, 'fast tracking' was commonly discussed in relation to the post-cardiac surgical patient. The term has a slightly differing meaning in different establishments, but it is always connected with the early weaning and extubation of patients after cardiac surgery. It may or may not refer to the earlier discharge from an intensive care/recovery area to a more progressive care area.

'Fast tracking' of patients has coincided with a change in the role of the nurse caring for cardiac surgical patients. To enable earlier weaning and extubation, nurses have undertaken the decision-making role that is traditionally the domain of medical staff. This has enabled nurses to become autonomous, and has assisted in the provision of more holistic care for patients. Not all patients are suitable for 'fast tracking' or early extubation. Now patients are generally older and sicker, and they may be more susceptible to myocardial ischaemia in the early postoperative period. The individual patient's condition must be weighed up against the continued improvements in all areas of surgery.

It may be possible to identify patients who can be fast tracked preoperatively, but many can only be identified postoperatively, with the main contraindications being evolving myocardial infarction or decompensated heart failure or both. Intraoperative proceedings are also important – prolonged cardiopulmonary bypass times or sustained hypothermia < 32°C are also factors that may prevent fast tracking.

Respiratory care required by patients after cardiac surgery therefore ranges from continuous mechanical ventilation to patients breathing spontaneously with no supplementary oxygenation but requiring breathing exercises. The nurse, who is constantly present, needs good knowledge and skill in the assessment of respiratory status, and should have an ability to analyse results of respiratory observations. They are assisted in their role by physiotherapists, who provide further respiratory assessment and advice.

The patient requiring mechanical ventilation

Most patients undergo a period of positive pressure ventilation, the length of which is determined by the condition of the patient, although 80% of patients should require only a short period of this support, i.e. up to 4 hours. A small percentage of patients may not require any positive pressure ventilation, but facilities for ventilation should be available. These patients have usually undergone atrial septal defect (ASD) repairs or are very young bypass graft recipients. Generally, the patients requiring longer periods of ventilation can be identified preoperatively, with assessment being based on the type of surgery required and the general physical condition preoperatively. Early extubation should be considered for all patients unless significant contraindications, such as multisystem dysfunction, persistence of impaired cardiac function, prolonged cardiopulmonary bypass with prolonged hypothermia or postoperative bleeding, are present. There are several complications associated with mechanical ventilation, which can be virtually eliminated with early extubation (Table 4.1).

Table 4.1 Complications of mechanical ventilation

Complication	Associated problem
Compromised airway	Aspiration
	Decreased clearance of secretions
	Predisposition to infection
Foreign body in the form of an	Tube kinked
endotracheal tube	Tube plugged
	Rupture of pyriform sinus
	Tracheal stenosis
	Tracheal malacia
	Right main-stem intubation
	Cuff failure
	Sinusitus (with nasal placement)
	Otitis media
	Laryngeal oedema
Ventilation – mechanical	Ventricular malfunction
	Hypoventilation
	Hyperventilation
	Tension pneumothorax
Ventilation – physiological	Water and sodium retention
	Left ventricular dysfunction – hypotension
	Stress ulcers
	Paralytic ileus
	Gastric distension

ET, endotracheal.

The nurse is responsible for ensuring that the ventilator is functioning properly before the patient's return from the operating room, and that equipment for emergency airway management in the event of mechanical failure is available and in working order. Standard ventilator settings are usually chosen with regard to the amount of supplementary oxygen, respiratory rate and tidal volume. Tidal volume is usually determined by the factor of 10 ml/kg of body weight. Upon the patient's return, the ventilator is attached to the patient's endotracheal (ET) tube, and the anaesthetist should ensure that the appropriate ventilator settings are chosen for the patient, based on the intraoperative and immediate postoperative assessment.

The ultimate aim of ventilation is to ensure adequate oxygenation. The initial effectiveness of ventilation in the delivery of oxygen can be determined by direct observation – watching the chest rise and fall. Auscultation of equal breath sounds is also recommended, but equal breath sounds have been reported even when the tube has migrated into the right bronchus. A chest radiograph is frequently advocated to ensure correct placement of the ET tube in addition to other invasive lines, but when short-term ventilation is planned this is not always requested. Endotracheal tubes are marked with a radio-opaque strip. Studies have shown that ET tubes are frequently malpositioned but this is more common after an emergency (Juniper and Gerrard, 1997). Observing the oxygen saturation (pulse oximetry) will demonstrate sufficient oxygen perfusion, but results should be treated cautiously in the hypothermic, shut-down and potentially anaemic patient. Arterial blood gases provide confirmation of the effectiveness of ventilation.

Continuous reading of oxygen saturation by pulse oximetry has become popular in recent years. It operates on the principles of Beer's law, which states that the concentration of an unknown solute dissolved in a solvent can be determined by light. Pulse oximetry works on the assumption that anything that pulses and absorbs red and infrared light between the light source and the light detector must be arterial blood. Its main function is to detect hypoxaemia, which occurs at a saturation of about 75% in normally perfused patients. As the brain is the most sensitive organ to oxygen depletion, the more obvious signs of hypoxia – visual and cognitive changes – will occur only when oxyhaemoglobin saturation falls to around 80–85% (Hanning and Alexander-Williams, 1995). Pulse oximetry is well tolerated by the sedated patient but can become easily dislodged in the confused or restless patient. The probe itself can exert a substantial amount of pressure on the digit to which it is attached and, without regular change in the position of the probe, ulcers similar to pressure sores can develop.

If a deteriorating oxygen saturation is detected, it is important that an arterial blood sample is taken for further analysis of the reasons. This blood sample is normally taken by the nurse at the bedside, via an arterial line. Table 4.2 indicates the normal values of arterial blood gases. Blood obtained from a vein in an extremity gives information about that extremity; it can be misleading if the metabolism in the extremity differs from the metabolism of the body as a whole. Venous samples from central lines can be taken and, if the mixed venous blood oxygen is low, problems with the lungs and circulation should be suspected and further investigations would be expected.

Arterial blood gases give a general overview of any acidosis/alkalosis and how well the patient is tolerating the ventilator and the prescribed mode. Although these results need to be acknowledged, it is common for

Table 4.2 Normal arterial blood gas values

pH	7.35–7.45
PaO_2	12 kPa
$PaCO_2$	4.5–6.1 kPa
Base excess	+2 to –2
Sodium bicarbonate	22–26 mmol/l
Saturation	99%
Acidosis occurs if pH < 7.35	
Alkalosis occurs if pH > 7.45	
If oxygen saturation < 70%, the sample is thought to be venous	

patients to demonstrate a metabolic acidosis (defined as a pH < 7.36, base excess (BE) < 2 mmol/l and sodium bicarbonate > 22 mmol/l), during the hypothermic phase of their recovery. There is an ongoing debate on the imbalance that should occur before corrective treatment in the form of intravenous sodium bicarbonate should commence. There is general agreement, however, that any acidosis should be on an improving trend before weaning and ultimately extubation occur.

Arterial blood gas analysis

Oxygen requirements

Blood gases with a low PaO_2 (arterial oxygen partial pressure) requires an improvement in oxygenation by increasing the intake of oxygen.

Blood gases with a high PaO_2 can present a risk of oxygen toxicity, and to reduce this possibility the inspired oxygen needs to be the lowest concentration possible, so the fraction of inspired oxygen (FIO_2) is decreased.

Ventilation control

Blood gases with a low $PaCO_2$ (partial pressure of arterial carbon dioxide) and a high pH generally indicate hyperventilation. To increase the $PaCO_2$, the minute volume needs to be decreased by decreasing either the respiratory rate or the tidal volume. The patient's condition will often indicate whether the respiratory rate or the tidal volume needs to be decreased; however, if high airway pressure is a problem, reduction in tidal volume would be ideal.

Blood gases with a high $PaCO_2$ and a low pH generally indicate hypoventilation. To remove the excess $PaCO_2$, the minute volume needs to be increased, by increasing the respiratory rate or tidal volumes. Again the condition of the patient should influence the choice but, by increasing the tidal volume, the airway pressures may increase, so a higher respiratory rate may be warranted.

When achieving adequate oxygenation, it is recommended that the arterial oxygen saturation (SaO_2) be maintained above 97%, although, when deciding limits, preoperative respiratory function must be considered, e.g. for a patient with a history of chronic obstructive airway disease (COAD), an SaO_2 of 94% may be desirable. Once the SaO_2 has reached the required level, it is necessary to reduce the amount of supplementary oxygen required to maintain this level, and a supplement of 40% oxygen is the gold standard to be reached before weaning of positive pressure ventilation is considered.

In assisting the patient to maintain adequate oxygen saturation, attention must be given to the maintenance of a clear airway, maintenance of a patent ET tube and correct functioning of the ventilator. Patients return from the operating room intubated, and the presence of an ET tube is essentially a foreign body, making the patient more susceptible to infection. The presence of an ET tube also hinders the functioning of the body's natural defence mechanism of the mucociliary esculator or mucous blanket. With this mechanism, inhaled foreign matter, bacteria and debris are transported in the mucus of the cilia moving them up towards the throat at a rate of 2 ml/min (Prakash et al., 1977).

Patency of the airway can be ensured by maintaining the correct placement and suctioning of the ET tube. Table 4.1 also lists the main complications of ET tubes. Figure 4.1 demonstrates the correct anatomical placement of an ET tube. The tip of the ET tube should lie between the thoracic inlet and 2.5 cm proximal to the carina. A useful way to find the correct location for the tip of the ET tube is to draw an imaginary line from the middle of the arch of the aorta (aortic knob) to the trachea. The lowest point of the aortic knob across the trachea marks the carina (Reading, 1994). To allow the tip to rest on the carina can result in difficulty in suctioning, causing barotrauma and inadequate ventilation. The inflated cuff should fill the tracheal lumen without distorting the lateral walls. The tube position may vary up to 4 cm depending on the position of the patient's neck. Once the correct placement is determined, the ET tube should be secured in position by tapes, which prevent movement of the tube but will not restrict venous return. Migration into the right bronchus can occur if the tube is incorrectly secured, which can be detected by absence of chest movement and breath sounds on the left side, and deteriorating arterial blood gases. Failure to detect this can lead to atelectasis of the left lung. Patients with an ET tube should ideally be nursed with the head raised slightly to overcome any impedance in venous return caused by the tapes.

To compensate for the devoid mucociliary esculator, ET suction can be performed (the mucociliary esculator system is the normal process whereby the cilia continually transport debris upwards in the trachea to be expelled as sputum or swallowed). Although proving a very effective and safe procedure, it can be extremely painful for the patient so it should not be performed without prior assessment of need. The introduction of a suction catheter into the respiratory tract prompts the natural cough reflex in the unsedated patient, and with inadequate analgesia after surgery this can prove very traumatic. ET tube suction should generally be performed only when:

- there are audible secretions
- chest sounds indicate secretions
- there are deteriorating arterial blood gases with increased airway pressures
- extubating.

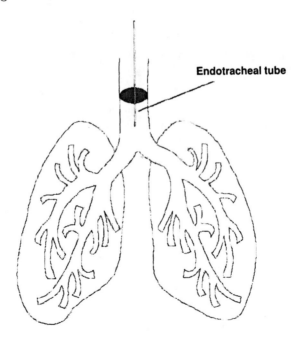

Figure 4.1 Correct placement of an endotracheal tube.

During a suctioning procedure, no more than −300 kPa of negative pressure should be used, and ideally only up to −200 kPa to minimise tracheal tissue damage. The size of the suction catheter should be the smallest possible size and should not exceed half the diameter of the ET tube. An equation for determining this is suggested in the following formula for measuring the maximum size of a suction catheter that should be used to suction down an ET tube:

ET tube size − 2 × 2.

The procedure should be clean, and gloves and goggles should be worn.

Ventilator settings

A malfunctioning ventilator is a very serious problem. Constant monitoring and hourly checks of the ventilator can minimise or spot potential problems. Low air volumes could indicate a leak in the ventilator circuit, whereas a high minute volume could indicate hyperventilation resulting from an increased spontaneous rate. Low airway pressures could indicate a leak, whereas high airway pressures may be influenced by positive end-expiratory pressure, but also be indicative of secretions, blockage and 'fighting' the ventilator.

Progressive weaning from mechanical ventilation and extubation is a priority goal in the postoperative period. Respiratory muscle atrophy begins 72–96 hours after full ventilation (MacIntyre, 1998) and weaning is thought to be more difficult in patients who have been ventilated for more than 48 hours (Hudak et al., 1986). Modern ventilators are very sophisticated pieces of equipment, which can be set according to the need(s) of the patient. The ventilatory mode refers to how the machine senses or signals the initiation of inspiration. The most common setting employed is volume-controlled ventilation in the form of intermittent mechanical ventilation (IMV) or synchronised intermittent mechanical ventilation (SIMV), which may or may not be supplemented by positive pressure support (PPS). SIMV and IMV provide a predetermined number of mandatory breaths per minute at a set tidal volume, but allow the patient to breathe spontaneously at his or her own respiratory rate and depth. The ultimate aim of the nurse is to wean a patient from the ventilator, so providing a mode that will allow patient-initiated breaths or spontaneous breaths is considered to be advantageous.

It is customary practice to add 5 cm of positive end-expiratory pressure (PEEP) to the ventilator. This substitutes for the loss of the physiological PEEP of normal breathing, which occurs in the presence of the ET tube. If oxygenation is poor, PEEP can be added in increments of 2.5–5 cm. However, increased PEEP may have adverse haemodynamic effects and mask the patient's haemodynamic parameters. PEEP at or above 10 cmH$_2$O may result in a higher central venous pressure (CVP) reading and a reduced cardiac output. In addition, high levels of PEEP may cause barotrauma.

The addition of positive pressure support ventilation (PSV) can ultimately help with weaning because it reportedly reduces muscle fatigue and helps the patient to synchronise with the ventilator. The PSV mode is triggered when the patient makes a spontaneous breath, and the ventilator delivers a preset airway pressure for the duration of inspiration.

Mechanical ventilation can cause several complications, which can be avoided with early weaning and extubation. The benefits of early weaning and extubation include the following:

- improved ciliary function and mucus transport in the respiratory tract
- reduced chance of a respiratory infection
- lower incidence of atelectasis or lobar collapse
- better cardiovascular function, with increased cardiac output and improved venous return.

Earlier extubation promotes earlier ambulation, quicker recovery and reduced costs.

When the patient shows signs of wakefulness, or is seen to make large amounts of spontaneous effort, i.e. tidal volume of 4–5 ml/kg, the weaning of ventilation should be considered. A tidal volume of less than 300 ml increases the risks of weaning failure. However, weaning by nursing staff should occur only if set criteria are met, unless the decision is made by medical staff. The use of predetermined criteria to determine a patient's readiness to wean has been shown to improve the success rates for patients after cardiac surgery. The criteria set for weaning may vary between establishments and there is a lot of controversy about the ideal procedure (Clochsey et al., 1997). Without protocols, patients would be weaned according to the clinician's personal experience and judgement. Table 4.3 demonstrates the criteria that the patient may be required to meet before weaning off ventilation.

Weaning can occur by a variety of methods.

Table 4.3 An example of criteria used in weaning off ventilation

---

- The patient is cardiovascularly stable. On occasions, it may be appropriate to initiate weaning on low doses of inotropes or vasodilators but the patient should be warmed centrally to 35°C and peripherally showing signs of warming
- Arterial blood gases are not showing a deteriorating trend, and electrolytes are within normal limits
- There is no significant respiratory depression from sedatives or opioids
- There is no evidence of respiratory distress
- Tidal volumes are > 300 ml
- If the patient's spontaneous rate is > 35, re-ventilation should be considered because chances of successful weaning are reduced, and therefore a further short period of ventilation should be considered
- The PaO_2 level is > 10 kPa on 40% oxygen
- Oxygen saturation should be > 95%
- Positive end-expiratory pressure or continuous positive airway pressure is down to 8 cmH_2O and/or PPS 12 cmH_2O (as measured at the endotracheal tube)
- Blood loss is < 400 ml in the first hour and < 100 ml thereafter

---

PPS, positive pressure support.

Spontaneous mode on the ventilator

This is advantageous for the use of alarms being triggered in the event of apnoea. However, even with the introduction of continuous positive airway pressure (CPAP) and PPS, it is hard work and a prolonged period may result in fatigue. Spontaneous mode is useful if weaning is to occur over a prolonged period. The amount of time the patient spends on the spontaneous mode can be increased progressively over a period of time, until the patient can be maintained on spontaneous mode continuously.

Reducing the ventilator rate

This is a gradual method of withdrawing ventilation, but still requires the patient to breathe against the ventilator. It can be effective after a short period of ventilation, but the gradual reduction in ventilatory support can be a slow method of weaning. There are advantages and disadvantages of using SIMV and reducing the ventilator rate during weaning. Typically, the ventilator breath rate is reduced by 2 breaths/min. With each decrease in the rate, the patient assumes more responsibility for his or her own ventilation in the form of spontaneous breaths, reducing the incidence of complications related to positive pressure ventilation. After each decrease, which may be at 30- to 60-min intervals, the patient's oxygen saturation is observed and arterial blood gas analysis performed.

Use of this method prevents weakening or atrophy of the pulmonary musculature because the patient uses these muscles during spontaneous breathing, although during weaning there is the potential of increasing the patient's effort to breathe as a result of inadequate ventilation and oxygenation. This method is not recommended in the weaning of patients after a prolonged period of ventilation.

In PPS, all breaths are initiated by the patient and supplemented with positive pressure ventilation. Providing PPS augments the patient's spontaneous tidal volume and decreases respiratory effort. It may be used alone or combined with IMV/SIMV. Used with SIMV, the spontaneous breaths are augmented between volume-controlled breaths. When the patient initiates inspiration, positive airway pressure or pressure support is delivered at a preset level. When the patient's inspiratory flow decreases below a specific level, pressure support ceases and exhalation occurs. PPS allows the patient to maintain his normal rate of breathing, length of time for inspiration, tidal volume and inspiratory flow rate. Combining SIMV and PPS benefits the patient who cannot tolerate reductions in the IMV mode of ventilation and will help the weaning process. The degree of respiratory support can be increased or decreased according to the patient's work of breathing. The main advantage of PPS is that it can overcome the imposed work of breathing, which affects respiratory muscle load. Imposed work of breathing refers to the additional resistance generated by the ET tube, ventilator, tubing circuit and humidifier, which must be overcome with spontaneous breathing.

Supplementary oxygen by a T piece

This method involves removing the patient from the ventilator and allowing him or her to breathe spontaneously via a T piece. It is a simple procedure and, if patients tolerate it, they can proceed to extubation. T-piece weaning, sometimes referred to as a spontaneous breathing trial, involves the use of a high-flow oxygen source attached to the intubated patient's ET tube via a T-shaped connector. Its value has been highlighted in patients who are on it short term, and it can be developed into a CPAP circuit if further support is needed. This appears to be the most popular method of weaning for patients who are ventilated in the short term and has been shown to be the quickest weaning method.

If the patient is for 'fast track' following cardiac surgery, extubation can usually occur after 30 minutes of weaning. Pulse oximetry has been shown to be more effective than arterial sampling in weaning to lower the percentage of inspired oxygen, because it allows continuous monitoring of the effects on the patient's oxygen saturation (Rotello et al., 1992). Criteria are usually available to guide the nurse in the decision-making process. Table 4.4 shows an extubation protocol. Traditional extubation criteria (bedside clinical parameters used to denote readiness for extubation) have remained broadly unchanged. Criteria usually include interpretation of vital capacity, inspired oxygen fraction and arterial blood gas analysis. Despite the complexity of some of the criteria, several studies suggest that successful extubation was statistically greater in patients who were described as having a normal level of consciousness and a strong cough reflex, supporting the effectiveness of clinical decision-making.

Before extubation, a system for providing supplementary oxygen should be available, and the process of extubation is easier if performed by two people. The patient should be assessed for bronchial secretions and, if necessary, ET suction should be given. Suction should be performed via the oropharynx to prevent any mucus or debris that has collected above the cuff from slipping down the trachea on cuff deflation. Extubation, as a procedure, has its complications; it is important that, on extubation, there are personnel in the vicinity who can perform emergency intubation. Table 4.5 lists the complications associated with extubation.

The patient requiring non-invasive respiratory support

After withdrawal of the ET tube, the patient should be encouraged to cough and expectorate any remaining mucus; encouraging patients to

Table 4.4 An example of criteria used in the extubation of patients

---

- The patient is exhibiting signs of spontaneous breathing
- The patient is cardiovascularly stable. Systolic blood pressure is > 95 mmHg on minimal inotropic support
- Patient should not show signs of respiratory distress
- There is no significant sign of respiratory depression
- PaO_2 is > 10 kPa on 40% oxygen
- Oxygen saturation should be 95% or above
- Arterial blood gases are not showing a deteriorating trend, and electrolytes are within normal limits
- The patient is comfortable, able to cough effectively and to clear secretions
- The patient is conscious, follows commands and is able to protect his or her airway (i.e. cough or gag reflex)
- Breath sounds are equal and clear

Table 4.5 The complications associated with extubation

Potential hazards during extubation
Laryngeal spasm
Regurgitation/inhalation
Vagal stimulation, dysrhythmias, cardiac arrest
Trauma

Potential complications following extubation
Hoarseness
Vocal cord paralysis
Dysphagia

speak will allow for the assessment of damage to the vocal cords. It is recommended that patients who were initially difficult to intubate should be extubated in the presence of an anaesthetist, or with the full agreement of medics, should laryngeal stridor occur, making re-intubation necessary.

Supplementary oxygen is usually administered via a facemask or nasal cannulae, and should usually be humidified. When oxygen is delivered at 3 l/min, there is no significant difference between the performance of these systems, although patients commonly tolerate nasal cannulae better (English and Brown, 1994). The upper airway normally warms, moistens and filters inspired gas. If this mechanism is bypassed for any length of time, then a means of artificial humidification is required. Inspired air is warmed and humidified by the naso-oropharynx to reach the upper airway with a relative humidity of about 90% and a temperature of 32–36°C. Humidification of inspired gas is required to preserve mucociliary and pulmonary function in most patients. In intubated patients (or those with a tracheostomy), the naso-orophyarnx is bypassed and the relative humidity falls to 50% or less. This presentation of dry, cold gases direct to the trachea has several adverse effects, which include an increase in mucus viscosity, reduced ciliary function, micro-atelectasis caused by obstruction of the small airways and large airway obstruction from tenacious sputum (Harrison et al., 1993). Sputum is a mucus secretion produced by the mucous membrane lining the respiratory tract. It is produced in response to inflammation, infection or congestive impairment of pulmonary function, and is the most significant postoperative complication following cardiac surgery.

Impairment of pulmonary function is another significant postoperative complication after cardiac surgery. On occasions, a patient may experience difficulty in expectorating tenacious secretions or sustain a degree of lobular collapse, when additional support mechanisms may be required. An initial strategy is to increase the amount of supplementary oxygen and humidification. It is normally only possible to achieve 40% oxygenation without the delivery of a high inspiratory flow, and where possible warm humidification should be used.

If lobular collapse does not resolve, a CPAP circuit should be used. This is a non-invasive respiratory support, which will be well tolerated by the cooperative patient. CPAP is commonly used for patients who have ineffective ventilation and oxygenation by increasing a patient's functional residual capacity, i.e. increasing the volume of air in the lungs at the end of expiration. CPAP exerts positive airway pressure throughout the entire respiratory cycle during spontaneous breathing. Typically, the amount of resistance used is between 2 and 20 cmH_2O, and patients exhale against this pressure. This back pressure re-expands and stabilises alveoli and helps to maintain patent airways. It can be delivered using a facial or nasal mask, or by ventilators attached to a tracheal tube. CPAP is useful in increasing PaO_2 levels postoperatively or to re-expand atelectatic lung tissue in adults. If used correctly, it will prevent the need for further ventilation. This increased ventilatory support will be enhanced by physiotherapy.

In contrast to CPAP, bilateral positive airway pressure (BiPAP) provides higher pressure during inspiration than during expiration, and can include a back-up respiratory rate with a fixed inspiratory and expiratory ratio. BiPAP is indicated for patients who require higher levels (> 100 cmH_2O) of inspiratory airway pressure to support ventilation.

The role of the physiotherapist is to prevent chest infections, encourage early mobilisation, and provide education and rehabilitation. Chest physiotherapy is not well defined but usually includes deep breathing exercises and adjuncts, positive manual techniques, coughing and suctioning, although in some patients methods used may provoke unwanted cardiorespiratory effects (Enright, 1992). In the long-term ventilated patients, techniques such as postural drainage, percussion and vibration may be beneficial, in conjunction with manual hyperinflation if copious secretions are present (Selsby and Jones, 1990). Prone positioning of the patient may improve oxygenation. Instilling saline at the top of the airway is not effective in loosening secretions, but can help to loosen dry secretions when instilled deeper into the bronchi, and ensures that a specimen is obtained for microbiological investigation.

In the non-ventilated patient, deep breathing aims to help airway clearance, improve respiratory muscle strength, and increase and maintain thoracic gas volume and rib-cage mobility. Thoracic expansion exercises are deep breathing, which emphasises inspiration and incorporates the concept of promoting collateral ventilation flow. Holding the breath at the end of inspiration promotes collateral flow. The inspiratory spirometer is an adjunct to physiotherapy and provides visual feedback on deep breathing. Three therapies – CPAP, positive expiratory pressure (PEP) and inspiratory resistance-PEP (IR-PEP) – may be used to supplement standard physiotherapy.

Patients who continue to experience difficulty in expectoration may require a mini-tracheostomy. Although this is not as radical as a tracheostomy, it is still invasive and subjects the patient to additional potential complications. To prevent patients experiencing difficulty in expectorating it is necessary to provide:

- saline nebulisers
- adequate analgesia.

Patients who experience uncontrolled pain will be reluctant to cough or deep breathe. Although this may not result in complications, it does predispose to chest infections and it is important that, while patients continue to expectorate, sputum is observed for discoloration and is sent for laboratory examination if greeny sputum is accompanied by raised temperatures.

Respiratory complications after cardiac surgery

Respiratory problems will result in a prolonged hospital admission. Vargas et al. (1993) suggest that 30% of patients will experience some respiratory complications by day 6 postoperatively.

Prolonged mechanical ventilation

Ventilatory complications are more likely to occur with a prolonged spell of mechanical ventilation or if there is a history of chest disease. This can occur as a direct result of a patient's respiratory function or as a result of cardiovascular instability, which requires an enforced period of ventilation. A patient should ideally be prepared in respect of not smoking and being clear of coughs and colds. The patient can very quickly become dependent on a ventilator and weaning can take several days. Patients who require long-term ventilation have a mortality rate of 30–40% (Scheinhorn et al., 1994).

Weaning failure is a multifactorial problem, and the withdrawal of ventilatory support is complicated by muscle fatigue (particularly respiratory muscles) and malnutrition, as well as general illness. Adequate nutrition and supplementary minerals are vital to provide energy for weaning. Inadequate nutrition can lead to the breakdown of respiratory muscles, and electrolyte disorders can impair the action of the diaphragm. Excessive carbohydrates may lead to hypercapnia and increased ventilatory drive. Hypercapnia may develop as a result of deterioration of the patient's condition (e.g. sepsis).

Factors identified as affecting the ability of a patient to be weaned include the following:

- the respiratory load and the capacity of the neurological system to cope with this load
- oxygenation
- cardiovascular performance
- psychological factors.

Respiratory load is determined by an increase in respiratory resistance from the patient's ET tube and airway, decrease in respiratory compliance and auto-PEEP, which is the trapping of air in the lungs to give a high PEEP. Fashioning of a tracheostomy can reduce respiratory resistance.

It is important to remember that weaning trials should not begin until a patient is receiving a low FIO_2 (< 40%). This generally suggests that the underlying condition is resolving with improved meeting of the target ventilation:perfusion ratio, which is affected by damaged alveolar tissue, e.g. infection. When lung tissue is recruited to perform gaseous exchange, oxygen levels will be decreasing.

Patients with poor left ventricular function are difficult to wean because the ventilator acts as a type of ventricular assist device. Reduced cardiac function will rely on the positive pressure created by the ventilator.

Nursing a person who is attempting to cope with a reduction in mechanical ventilation is reliant on the provision of encouragement to the patient, and the early recognition of any inability to cope with weaning. In addition, as well as regular ET suction, attention must be paid to the prevention of pressure to the mouth and facial tissue that can arise from the ET tube and the securing tapes. The tapes should be changed on a regular basis, particularly in the presence of excessive saliva, but on at least a daily basis. The ET tube, despite being secured by tapes, tends to migrate to the corner of the mouth, and this then creates pressure on the lips. The tube should therefore be repositioned in the mouth at least once every 24 hours.

Respiratory failure

Impairment of pulmonary function is one of the most significant complications after bypass surgery. Many factors may increase the likelihood of respiratory failure, including respiratory depressant drugs, high left atrial pressure, atelectasis, pulmonary microembolism, increase in extravascular lung water, and the use of single or bilateral internal mammary artery grafts. Signs of respiratory distress include the following: rapid shallow breathing; reduced arterial oxygen saturation; increase of arterial carbon dioxide levels; reduced tidal volumes; use of accessory muscles; increased heart rate; and reduced level of consciousness.

Respiratory infection

The incidence of infection is increased if prolonged ventilation occurs. It takes approximately 24 hours for bacteria in the oral cavity to migrate down the respiratory tract in the intubated patient, even when scrupulous oral care is given. Once a respiratory infection occurs in a ventilated patient, weaning will be delayed until the infection is controlled by antibiotics and supplementary oxygen requirements are reduced. The development of pneumonia is thought to delay postoperative discharge by 11 days (Weintraub et al., 1989).

Pneumonia

Distinguishing pneumonia from other complications by radiology alone can be difficult, particularly when bilateral changes are present. The clinical state of the patient should always be considered in conjunction with radiographic findings and other investigations. Prone positioning, particularly for patients suspected of acute respiratory distress syndrome (ARDS), has shown favourable results. This could be advantageous in mobilising secretions, but can be a consideration only when the patient becomes haemodynamically stable.

Bronchospasm

Bronchospasm can occur at the termination of surgery, and may hinder sternal closure or mechanical ventilation. Patients with known asthma should have salbutamol inhalers recommenced after surgery. Bronchospasm can also occur after extubation. It should be treated with the appropriate β agonists, theophylline derivatives or steroids.

Pulmonary oedema

This can be divided into cardiogenic (haemodynamic) and non-cardiogenic (permeability). The latter is most commonly the result of ARDS. Factors such as upper lobe venous enlargement, perihilar and basal distribution, enlargement of the vascular pedicle, and cardiomegaly, have been proposed as indicative of a cardiogenic cause.

Tracheostomy

Although this can cause complications, it is usually electively required when prolonged ventilation has occurred for 10 days, unless weaning is to occur within 14 days. Creating a tracheostomy will ultimately make weaning easier, by reducing dead space and increasing patient comfort (enabling reduced sedation), and avoid the need for reintubation if extubation fails. However, the risk of infection, both respiratory and in the sternal wound, is increased. Secretions from a tracheostomy can not only invade the insertion sites of invasive lines around the neck, but also come into contact with the sternal surgical wound.

Atelectasis

Causes of lobar collapse include malposition of the ET tube and mucus plugging. More frequently, peripheral airway plugging with secretions results in peripheral subsegmental atelectasis, seen as thin band shadows usually present in the mid and lower zones of the lung. Minor degrees of atelectasis are extremely common following surgery, occurring in up to 85% of patients after thoracic surgery and 20% after extrathoracic procedures.

Any ventilated patient is prone to atelectasis. This can be prevented by turning/repositioning a patient at regular intervals and physiotherapy. A chest radiograph may confirm clinical diagnosis. Once it occurs, the effects can be improved by the use of PEEP/CPAP and turning the patient. A degree of pulmonary atelectasis, particularly of the left lower lobe, is very common after cardiac surgery, but usually responds to physiotherapy

Pneumothorax

This is an identified complication of mechanical ventilation, but can also occur during the insertion of central lines. The normal indications on a radiograph of absent lung markings, increased transradiancy and visible visceral pleura may be obscured in a radiograph taken in the supine position. Depression of one hemidiaphragm and mediastinal shift away from the affected side suggest a tension pneumothorax. After discharge, pleural effusion is one of the most common causes of a patient requiring readmission to hospital (Johnson, 2000).

Anxiety

Patients who require mechanical ventilation often have anxieties related to their dependence on the machine, as well as the tubing, alarms and communication barriers. Unaddressed, these concerns may delay the patient's weaning from a ventilator. Mechanical ventilation can affect the patient's sensory input and this can be aggravated by the use of sedation and muscle relaxing agents (see Chapter 6).

References

Clochsey JM, Burns SM, Shekleton ME et al. (1997) Volunteers in participatory sample survey of weaning practices. Third national study group on weaning from mechanical ventilation. *Crit Care Nurse* 17(2): 72–8.

English I, Brown C (1994) Recovery nursing: oxygen mask or nasal catheter? An analysis *Nursing Standard* 8: 27–31.

Enright S (1992) Cardiorespiratory effects of chest physiotherapy. In: Rinnie M, ed., *Intensive Care Britain*. London: Greycoat Publications, pp. 118–23.

Hanning CD, Alexander-Williams JM (1995) Pulse oximetry: a practical review. *BMJ* 311: 367–70.

Harrison DA, Breen DP, Harris NP (1993) The performance of two intensive care humidifiers at high gas flows. *Anaesthesia* 48: 902–5.

Higgins TL (1992) Pro: early endotracheal extubation is preferable to late extubation in patients following coronary artery surgery. *J Cardiothorac Vasc Anaesth* 6: 488–93.

Hudak CM, Gallo BM, Lohr T (1986) *Critical Care Nursing. A holistic approach*. London: Lippincott.

Johnson K (2000) Use of telephone follow up for post cardiac surgery patients. *Intensive Crit Care Nursing* 16: 144–50.

Juniper MC, Gerrard CS (1997) The chest x-ray in intensive care. *Care of the Critically Ill* 13(5): 198–200.

Lefemine AA, Harken DE (1966) Post operative care following open heart operations: routine use of controlled ventilation. *J Thorac Cardiovasc Surg* 52: 207–16.

MacIntyre NR (1998) Weaning from mechanical ventilatory support: volume assisting intermittent breaths versus pressure assisting every breath. *Respir Care* 33(2): 121–5.

Prakash O, Johnson B, Meij S et al. (1977) Criteria for early extubation after intracardiac surgery in adults. *Anaesth Analg* **56**: 703–8.

Reading MC (1994) Chest x-rays, tubes, catheters and wires. *Aust Crit Care J* **7**(4): 24–9.

Rotello LC, Warren J, Jastremski MS, Milewski A (1992) A nurse directed protocol using pulse oximetry to wean mechanically ventilated patients from toxic oxygen concentrations. *Chest* **102**: 1833–5.

Scheinhorn DJ, Artinian BM, Catlin JC (1994) Weaning from prolonged mechanical ventilation: the experience of a regional weaning centre. *Chest* **105**: 534–9.

Selsby D, Jones JG (1990) Some physiological and clinical aspects of chest physiotherapy. *Br J Anaesth* **12**: 621–31.

Vargas F, Cukier A, Terra-Filho M, Hueb W, Teixeira L, Light RW (1993) Influence of atelectasis on pulmonary function after coronary artery bypass grafting. *Chest* **104**: 434–7.

Weintraub W, Jones C, Craver J, Guyton R, Cohen C (1989) Determinants of prolonged length of hospital stay after coronary bypass surgery. *Circulation* **8**(2): 276–84.

CHAPTER 5

Maintaining a patient's haemodynamic stability

The patient's cardiovascular function requires careful monitoring during the initial period of the recovery, and definitely during the intensive care phase of the recovery. How quickly monitoring is discontinued depends on the stability of the patient. Several measurements should be considered concurrently in assessing the cardiovascular status, but for the purposes of clarity these will initially be identified as separate readings.

Heart rate

The numerous monitoring devices are variously three-, four- or five-electrode monitors. All monitors require use of a positive and negative electrode. Monitors that need three electrodes use positive, negative and ground electrodes, which are placed in the right arm, left arm and left leg position on the chest (Figure 5.1). A fourth electrode is in the right leg position, and the fifth can be placed in any of the six chest lead positions on the chest (Figure 5.2). The lead usually chosen for monitors is lead II, but modified chest lead 1 (MCL1) is most helpful for differentiating dysrhythmias. The choice of monitoring lead should be based on the arrhythmia most likely to occur and be clinically significant to the patient.

Cardiac monitors are useful only if the information that they provide is observed by setting alarms and interpreted by competent individuals. Multi-lead monitoring is better than single lead monitoring. Although bedside ECG traces can signify dysrhythmias, true diagnosis of an arrhythmia can be achieved only by recording a 12-lead ECG. Obviously, if the rhythm has resulted in a cardiac arrest, resuscitation is the priority.

The optimum heart rate should be maintained in order to achieve an adequate cardiac output, but when deciding on the optimum the

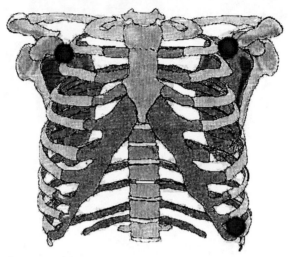

Figure 5.1 The placement of three electrodes for cardiac monitoring.

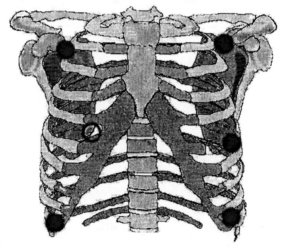

Figure 5.2 The placement of five electrodes for cardiac monitoring.

patient's preoperative condition should be referred to. Most patients will remain in a sinus rhythm, although this may occasionally present as a bradycardia (rate < 60 beats/min) or a tachycardia (rate > 100 beats/ min). These slow or rapid rates generally require correction only if they have a detrimental effect on cardiac output.

Cardiac dysrhythmias are associated with complications postoperatively, some of which may be temporary and correctable by chemical means (i.e. drugs), although some are potentially lethal but correctable by mechanical means. These postoperative arrhythmias may occur as a result of surgical technique, the technique of myocardial protection, and electrolyte and acid–base imbalances. The nurse has a responsibility to recognise abnormal and normal ECG tracings and initiate treatment to prevent patients from becoming cardiovascularly unstable.

Monitoring continues for 24 hours, and is then discontinued based on a general assessment of the patient. If all normal cardiovascular parameters are met, with no support, and the patient has not displayed dysrhythmias, the monitoring can be discontinued. As a result of the risk of ischaemia occurring during anaesthesia, a 12-lead ECG should be routinely recorded in the first 24 hours following surgery and again after 3 days to determine myocardial re-perfusion. Once monitoring has been discontinued, it is still important to record the patient's pulse regularly until discharge. This should be taken manually so that irregularities can be detected.

The incidence of cardiac dysrhythmias is 10–40% (Butler et al., 1993) and the dysrhythmias commonly seen can be classified as atrial or ventricular, the more common being listed in Table 5.1.

Atrial fibrillation

This is a very commonly occurring dysrhythmia; it is not unique to cardiac surgery and can be identified in most of the monitoring leads. Patients experiencing atrial fibrillation (AF) preoperatively are more likely to continue in this rhythm postoperatively. It is common in patients following coronary artery bypass grafts (CABGs), occurring in 4–50% of cases (Kolvekar et al., 1997), and may be a result of diffuse myocardial ischaemia or hypothermic surgery. In AF, there is a complete absence of coordinated atrial systole. It is characterised on the ECG by the absence of consistent p waves before each QRS complex. Although this dysrhythmia may be transient and self-correcting and does not generally affect the long-term outcome of surgery, treatment is imperative because there is an increasing awareness that AF is a major cause of embolic events which, in 75% of cases, are complicated by cerebrovascular accidents.

To prevent this devastating complication, treatment should be commenced on recognising AF. On occasions, restarting β blockers in the postoperative period may control the incidence and severity of AF. Treatment has traditionally been in the chemical form of digoxin, but this has the effect of lowing the heart rate rather than reversing the rhythm, and long-term use can lead to toxicity; its effectiveness is influenced by a

Table 5.1 Common rhythms and dysrhythmias

Sinus rhythm	Will be displayed by most patients. The rate ranges from 60 to 100 beats/min and is regular
Sinus tachycardia	Ranges from 100 to 160/min and is a response for increased cardiac output. A regular rhythm that may occur in the presence of pain, fever, fear, anxiety, congestive heart failure or hypovolaemia, or may be drug induced. Treat the cause and the rate will reduce
Sinus bradycardia	Regular rhythm of a rate < 60 beats/min. Causes include increased cranial pressure, cervical or mediastinal tumours, anaesthesia, hypoxia and hypothermia. Treatment includes oxygen, warming and intravenous atropine or pacing
Sinus arrest/sinus pause	Failure of impulse formation in the sinus node. The rhythm is irregular, rate can vary or become sinus bradycardia. Causes include digitalis toxicity, carotid sensitivity and increased vagal tone. Treated by intravenous atropine of pacing
Premature atrial contractions (PACs)	A premature impulse arising in the atria, but not from the sinoatrial node. Causes include anxiety, hypoxia, electrolyte imbalance and nicotine use. Rhythm is irregular. Treatment: oxygen, correct electrolyte imbalance and treat pain
Atrial fibrillation	Rapid, irregular atrial impulses and ineffective atrial contraction. Rate varies from 160 to 180 beats/min, but is grossly irregular. Causes: hypotension, post-cardiac surgery hypoxia, pulmonary embolism. Treatment includes oxygen, cardioversion, digoxin and warfarin
Atrial flutter	Abnormal atrial excitation: rate regular at 200-33 beats/min. Causes include open heart surgery, hypoxia, mitral or tricuspid disease. Treatment is by cardioversion, rapid atrial pacing or antiarrhythmic medication
Premature ventricular contraction	Ectopic beat from the ventricles. Causes include hypokalaemia, hypercalaemia, adrenaline and fever. Treatment is required only if the patient is symptomatic

patient's urea and electrolytes. Patients would require concurrent anti-coagulation therapy, and life-long follow-up, which may add further strain to an over-stretched health service. Amiodarone may also be commenced intravenously, and once a therapeutic level has been achieved therapy could continually orally.

Patients who are prescribed digoxin should be given a loading dose intravenously or orally. Before the initial administration, the serum potassium should be checked because low potassium can potentiate the effects of digoxin and the patient could become bradycardic or even asystolic.

The effectiveness of treatment can be determined by simultaneously recording the apex and radial pulse. There is a danger when patients are monitored or when mechanical methods are employed to record blood pressure that deficits and possibly irregularities are undetected.

Emphasis in treatment is now directed at cardioversion. This is an elective process of applying a synchronised direct current shock to the chest to revert the patient into a sinus rhythm. This is a safe procedure, providing that consent is gained from the patient and the patient's airway is protected during a period of sedation. The energy required for cardioversion is the focus of debate, but energy from 50 J has been used successfully to restore sinus rhythm. Late development of AF may require a 6-week course of anticoagulants before elective cardioversion. AF is one of the most frequent reasons for a patient's readmission to hospital in the first 4 weeks after surgery (Johnson, 2000).

Atrial fibrillation alone does not require patient monitoring once treatment has been initiated, and once it has been controlled it should not seriously impede recovery.

Heart block

Heart block may complicate an aortic valve replacement (AVR) because of oedema, haemorrhage, suturing or débridement near to the conduction system, which lies adjacent to the base of the right coronary cusp. It can be identified in any chest lead that displays clear p waves and QRS complexes. Epicardial atrioventricular (AV) pacing may be required for several days. If heart block persists for more than 1 week, during which time oedema or haemorrhage should subside, placement of a permanent pacemaker is usually considered. Disturbances of the AV conduction are also fairly frequent after a CABG, with an incidence of approximately 25%. The incidence is believed to be higher after the use of cold potassium cardioplegia and pacing wires may not be inserted after non-bypass surgery. Most disturbances resolve within 24–48 hours.

Epicardial pacing

Pacing wires are generally inserted before the termination of cardiopulmonary bypass so that they are available, if needed, to maintain a heart rate that will provide an adequate cardiac output and ensure AV synchrony. Insertion is easier while the patient is on cardiopulmonary bypass, when the lungs are deflated and out of the way of the right atrium. Pacing wires attached to the atrium are universally placed to the right of the sternum, ventricular wires to the left (Figure 5.3). The wires are usually removed on postoperative day 4 or 5 unless in use.

The fixation coil of the pacing wire can be positioned on the atrium or the ventricle. The fixation coil and the electrode are pulled into the myocardium with the needle at the end of the lead. When the electrode and a portion of the coil are in position, the remaining coil and needle are cut and removed. A scored Keith needle is used to bring the wire out through the chest wall. Some wires are positioned at the base of the sternotomy skin incision. The needle is broken at the second scored section, and the wire is connected immediately into an external generator or into a joining cable that is connected to the generator.

In some cases, one ventricular wire may be placed on the ventricle for pacing when a green needle is used as a second ground wire. The electrode needs a negative and positive pole, so that the current can flow between the pulse generator and the heart. The negative pole does the pacing, the positive pole serves as the ground. The pacing threshold is the minimum amount of energy (in milliamps) that will stimulate an electrical response in the heart. On return from the operating room, if a patient requires pacing, the threshold should be determined and doubled to allow for the subsequent development of oedema around the operation site and the build-up of fibrous tissue around the electrode. The sensitivity threshold is the number of millivolts needed to inhibit the pacemaker from firing.

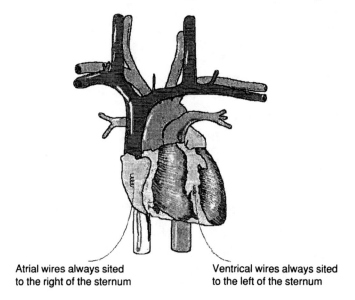

Atrial wires always sited   Ventrical wires always sited
to the right of the sternum   to the left of the sternum

Figure 5.3 Internationally agreed standard for the placement of epicardial wires.

Cardiac output is the product of stroke volume and heart rate. The optimum heart rate for patients returning from cardiac surgery is 90 beats/min. Temporary pacing can be used to stabilise and increase cardiac output. The most common indications for pacing after cardiac surgery are:

- complete heart block
- atrial fibrillation with low ventricular rate
- bradycardia.

If a patient presents with an abnormal heart rate of less than 60 beats/min, and is not in sinus rhythm, pacing should commence.

Pacing boxes are commonly single chamber but are increasingly becoming dual chamber. Single chamber suggests that only one chamber at any one time can be paced. However, loss of the atrial contraction results in a loss of 33% of ventricular filling (atrial kick). The ability to pace both atria and ventricle (sequential pacing) improves cardiac output.

The usual temporary pacing modes used are the following:

- VVI: demand ventricular pacing
- AAI: demand atrial pacing
- DDI/DDD: demand dual-chamber pacing
- AOO/VOO: fixed rate pacing (not frequently used).

Fixed pacing can be dangerous, and demand is the ideal way to pace the ventricle. Fixed pacing can be used in bradycardia, but problems could occur if the inherent rate returns, and this type of pacing now appears outdated.

The following parameters need setting:

- Sensitivity: the strength of the electrical activity that the pacemaker interprets as an atrial or ventricular pulse
- Output: the strength of the pulse delivered by the pacemaker (after surgery the amount required is determined and doubled to compensate for oedema as a result of surgery)
- Mode, i.e. demand/fixed rate: atrial, ventricular or dual.

Pacing boxes need to deliver enough energy to cause a contraction with enhanced quantity or time (sequential). On the traditional boxes, only the quantity of the contraction can be influenced.

Care of epicardial wires

It has been suggested that gloves should be worn at all times when pacing wires are being handled to prevent stray shocks passing through the wires, resulting in patients receiving microshocks. These shocks may not be evident on an ECG, but may be sufficient to cause ventricular fibrillation (VF) in a patient with an irritable myocardium.

Patients requiring pacing should be nursed on a cardiac monitor to allow for pacemaker function to be assessed, by the absence or presence of pacing spikes. If only one pacing wire is *in situ*, a sterile needle should be easily accessible around the patient's bed area.

If pacing wires are not in use, they should be wrapped in dry gauze and taped lightly to the chest wall. The contents of the gauze should be labelled for easy identification should pacing need to be commenced, particularly if other dressings are in place. If pacing is in progress, it is important that no traction is placed on the wires. The box and attached cable should be secure. Caution should be taken when moving patients who are connected to a pacemaker generator to prevent disruption of the connections or dislodgement of the wires.

Mediastinal bleeding can occur if rigid pacing wires are placed too close to bypass grafts, shearing them by intermittent contact during ventricular contractions. The pacemaker settings in relation to rate and output should be documented on a daily basis.

The wires are usually removed on postoperative day 4 or 5, sometimes earlier. Patients on warfarin should have their international normalised ratio (INR) checked to ensure that it is within the therapeutic range. Patients with a high INR should have the result relayed to medical staff. The patients should lie in the semi-recumbent position, and should remain on bedrest for a minimum of 30 min after removal of the pacing wire(s) to facilitate observation. The patients should be kept under observation for 1 h, i.e. they should not be allowed home immediately after removal of the wires. There is a risk of sudden haemorrhage when temporary pacing wires are removed. Bleeding occurs secondary to laceration of the myocardium, nearby blood vessels or an adjacent bypass graft (Johnson et al., 1993). If chest drains are present, a sudden increase in drainage will occur. However, pacing wires are often removed after mediastinal drainage tubes have been taken out, and rapid tamponade can occur because blood remains confined to the pericardium. Pericardial tamponade can occur within 60 min, after removal of pacing wires. Pericardiocentesis may be attempted, but mediastinal exploration in the patient's ward or the operating room may be needed to repair the tamponade.

Some patients may return from the operating room without epicardial pacing wires. On these occasions, if a patient becomes bradycardic, an isoprenaline infusion can be commenced or external pacing can be instituted.

Ventricular ectopics

The myocardium may be irritable from handling or the effects of the bypass machine after surgery. This may occasionally be identified by the presence of occasional or multiple ectopics. Although these may be a precursor to a more sinister rhythm, they may also be indicative of hypokalaemia, which is often present after surgery but which can be controlled with potassium supplements. Multiple ectopics may deteriorate into ventricular tachycardia or ventricular fibrillation.

Research demonstrates that leads V1 and V6 (or bipolar equivalents MCL1 and MCL6) are the best leads for differentiating wide QRS complexes (Jackson, 1998). Incorrect placement of invasive lines, such as central lines or pulmonary artery catheters, can also result in ventricular ectopics.

Ventricular tachycardia

When this occurs, it can be described as pulseless (cardiac arrest) or life-sustaining. It is advantageous to reverse this rhythm at the earliest opportunity. This may be achieved chemically or mechanically. Chemical agents can be lidocaine (lignocaine) or amiodarone, whereas elective cardioversion is a mechanical treatment.

Ventricular fibrillation

This is life-threatening and the only successful treatment is defibrillation, although precordial thump has been shown to be effective if applied at a witnessed event. This is commonly identified as a re-perfusion rhythm. If ventricular fibrillation is not recognised and treated early, the rhythm deteriorates into asystole from which the chances of successful resuscitation are limited.

The incidence of ventricular and atrial arrhythmias diminishes rapidly in the early in-hospital phase of the recovery, but as many as 15% of patients may continue to experience them until the time of discharge. These patients usually require only short-term (4–8 weeks), post-discharge treatment for the arrhythmias. Arrhythmias that persist after this time require special investigation, and are best suited to the skills of the cardiologist.

Temperature

During the operation patients are likely to become hypothermic either therapeutically or as a result of environmental cooling, so an initial aim on a patient's return is to assist him or her to gain a normal body temperature at around 37°C. Re-warming in the intensive care setting is typically a haemodynamically vulnerable time for the patient. Re-warming while on bypass significantly reduces the time lost on the unit to re-warming interventions which must be given priority over the reduction of ventilator support and extubation. Before leaving the operating room, the patient's body core is warmed to 35°C, but the body shell remains cold and, during the transfer back to the ward/recovery bay, the body core loses heat to the larger body shell and to the environment. This results in a drop in core temperature, and some patients are admitted back to the intensive care with a core temperature of less than 35°C.

Some degree of active re-warming may be required and interventions should be started when a baseline measurement has been achieved. Continuous monitoring of core body temperature is easily obtained from a rectal probe. The peripheral temperature provides an indication of cardiac output. Once a core temperature has reached 36°C, peripheral warming should start, in order to achieve a peripheral temperature of no more than 2°C lower than the core temperature. Failure could be a reflection of a compromised cardiac output. A peripheral probe is usually placed on a big toe and, if the patient has undergone bypass grafts using the saphenous vein as a donor site, the unaffected limb should be monitored. When an adrenaline (epinephrine) infusion is in progress, or the patient has been on atenolol preoperatively, the toe may not give a true indication of peripheral re-warming as a result of vasoconstriction. It is important that, in addition to monitoring the temperature gradient (i.e. core and peripheral temperature), assessment of the extent of peripheral warming by touch should also be carried out.

There are several consequences of prolonged hypothermia.

Shivering

Post-anaesthetic shivering is an attempt to generate heat, and may occur during re-warming. Body movements increase, the muscles become tense and energy is used to produce heat. Oxygen consumption can rise by 400–500%. The metabolic rate, carbon dioxide production and myocardial activity all increase. Shivering increases both blood viscosity and the risks of disseminated intravascular coagulation, and arterial oxygen saturation, mixed venous saturation and glycogen stores all decrease. Shivering should be abolished as soon as possible to avert increased metabolic demands and discomfort, and this can be achieved by the administration of 25 mg pethidine intravenously.

Re-warming shock

If peripheral re-warming occurs before central warming and promotes vasodilatation, cold, acidotic blood is returned to the heart and increases myocardial depression. It may also occur during re-warming if circulating volume is inadequate and vigilant haemodynamic monitoring is imperative to avoid re-warming shock.

Impaired immunity

Hypothermia may impair immunity. Collagen formation at the incision site demonstrates poor wound healing, and loss of nitrogen and protein increases the risk of both wound infection and prolonged recovery.

Impaired liver and pancreas

Hypothermia impairs hepatic and pancreatic function, reducing the release of insulin and uptake of glucose. It also increases serum glucose, resulting in circulating hyperglycaemia. If insulin is administered while the patient is hypothermic (i.e. core temperature > 35°C), there can be a re-entry of glucose as normothermia is restored, resulting in hypoglycaemia.

Acidosis

Re-warming that occurs too rapidly can be detrimental, because acidosis that has accumulated in the stagnant blood in the periphery will return to the heart during re-warming. A drop in blood pH occurs because of the sudden increase in lactic acid concentration, resulting in metabolic acidosis. Systemic acidosis depresses the functional activity of all vital organs.

Dysrhythmias

A slow heart and unusual QRS complexes are common during hypothermia. The incidence of cardiac arrest increases with decreasing temperatures. Atrial fibrillation, asystole and pulseless electrical activity (PEA) may occur.

Impaired kidney function

Hypothermia initiates a cold diuresis as a result of suppression of antidiuretic hormone secretion. This results in increased urinary output and water loss, leading to hypovolaemia. During the period of hypothermia, acute tubular necrosis and renal failure may occur.

High potassium levels

Alterations in the sodium/potassium pump may result in increased potassium levels, but hypokalaemia may follow during re-warming. A high potassium level (> 10 mmol/l) is often seen as a predictor of non-survival. The white cell count may be elevated, but it is not usually associated with infection.

Patient re-warming

There are several strategies available to assist patient re-warming:

• passive re-warming
• active surface warming
• active core warming.

Passive re-warming

Warmed blankets

While the patient is in the operating room, the bed and blankets can be warmed. This may help to reduce the effect of 'after drop', but it does not really contribute to active re-warming.

Space blanket

These were introduced by the armed services for survival purposes, before their introduction to the hospital environment. They work on the principle that heat is reflected back to assist in warming. There is debate on how effective they are when applied directly to a peripherally shut-down and cold patient. In addition, they may retain cold and cause the patient to sweat, so it is advisable to place a blanket or sheet against the patient. In these patients, peripheral temperature may decrease until the core temperature has warmed fully and only then does the peripheral temperature start to warm.

Active surface re-warming

Re-warming can occur by mechanical means using equipment designed for the purpose. A blanket that has warm air circulating through it (warmed forced air) is laid directly on top of the patient. Such blankets are effective, although while in use the patient must be carefully monitored to ensure that thermal burns do not occur. Rapid re-warming could result in haemodynamic instability so a combination of methods may be used, the method chosen depending on the equipment available or the initial body temperature. Patients with a normal body temperature but who are peripherally cold may not require aggressive re-warming. With any of these techniques, as a patient warms the amount of re-warming required should be reduced: i.e. turn the temperature down on the re-warming device, pull back any blankets.

Active core re-warming

This is when a bypass machine is used to warm the patient. Once the patient has achieved normal temperature, which should occur before weaning from ventilation, continual monitoring may be discontinued, although it may be prolonged in the presence of an adrenaline infusion or an intra-aortic balloon pump. Temperature overshoot has also been reported in the postoperative period. The rapid increase in core temperature is caused by the body's inability to lose heat as a result of surface vasoconstriction induced by hypothermia. This may warrant therapeutic cooling in the form of tepid sponging and rectal paracetamol. Elevated temperatures increase metabolic oxygen requirements, at a time when blood flow to the vital organs is already compromised. In an effort to avoid this, active internal and external re-warming should be discontinued before a temperature of 36.4°C is reached. A pyrexia occurring after a 48-hour period is usually connected to an infection.

For the remainder of the patient's stay, the temperature should be monitored, the frequency depending on the surgery performed. A raised temperature at any stage may be indicative of an infection, which could be respiratory, urinary or of the wound, and relevant swabs should be sent to determine diagnosis and treatment as required. A raised temperature observed in patients after a valve replacement may have a more sinister implication, and endocarditis may be suspected and splinter haemorrhages under the finger nails evident. When an elevated temperature occurs in patients who have had valve surgery, blood cultures must be taken. If endocarditis does occur, this will warrant a prolonged course of antibiotics with a prolonged hospital stay or reoperation. All patients will demonstrate a temperature variance in a 24-hour period, but a pyrexia occurring in the early evening is thought to be a reliable measure.

There are now various methods of monitoring temperature and it is important that the equipment is used correctly to ensure accuracy of information.

Central venous pressure

The central venous pressure (CVP) reflects the volume of blood returning to the heart, which exerts a pressure on the walls of the right atrium. It is maintained by vascular capacity, circulating blood volume and cardiac pump action. The tip of the catheter should be intrathoracic and intravascular, and not intracardiac (Figure 5.4). The central line is usually inserted by the internal jugular vein when the risk of complications, i.e. malposition

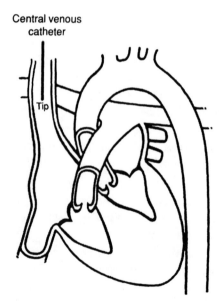

Figure 5.4 The correct placement of a central venous catheter. Reproduced with kind permission of Datascope Medical Co. Ltd.

or pneumothorax, is suggested to be less than 3% (Gray et al., 1992). Extravascular siting may lead to pleural effusion or mediastinal widening, intracardiac positions increase the risk of cardiac dysrhythmias or perforation, and extravascular positioning may lead to incorrect measurement of CVP. At the tip of the central line there is little difference between systolic and diastolic pressures, so the CVP is measured as a mean pressure.

Central lines can alternatively be sited in the subclavian vein. The subclavian site is more secure and the lack of mechanical movement reduces the chance of malposition. However, although this site may be the most preferable, it is often contraindicated in those requiring mechanical ventilation because of an increased risk of pneumothorax and subsequent tension pneumothorax from positive pressure ventilation. The internal jugular vein is considered only for short-term use.

Generally, there is an overestimation of the value of the CVP reading, particularly when taken in isolation. When positive end-expiratory pressure (PEEP) is applied to the ventilatory circuit, the CVP will rise, and the effects of this are particularly noticeable at levels greater than 10 cmH$_2$O. A fall in the CVP is perceived to indicate a moderate hypovolaemia, which may be precipitated by vasodilatation and peripheral warming. A patient who is hypovolaemic may appear to have a normal pressure caused by the inclusion of PEEP. A consequent rise in CVP may give rise to concerns over fluid overload or cardiac tamponade. A CVP can therefore be used as a guide to determine the severity of fluid loss, to measure when too much has been administered and to ascertain cardiac instability. A more accurate reflection of cardiac function and volume can be determined from pulmonary artery catheters.

Patients who have required the use of an extracorporeal circulation during surgery frequently reveal marked hypovolaemia, in spite of a highly positive fluid balance. This is thought to be the result of transient microvascular damage and extravascular fluid shift. Therefore, volume replacement to achieve haemodynamic stability may cause fluid overload and congestive heart failure. Colloids are widely used in the replacement of fluid volume, but doubt remains about their benefit. Different colloids vary in their molecular weight and, therefore, the length of time they remain in the circulatory system varies.

Triple-lumen catheters allow for continual monitoring of CVP and administration of large-volume fluids, irritant drugs, etc. When assessing the haemodynamic status, attention must be paid to the positioning of the patient. If the patient is in the lateral position (on the right side), the vena cava may be compressed, particularly in the obese patient, with subsequent reduction in pre-load. The reference point for aligning the right atrium in the measurement of CVP may be one of the following positions: the sternal angle, which is a point directly above the right atrium when the patient is lying flat (CVP normal value 0–4 mmHg) or, alternatively, the fourth intercostal space in the middle of the axilla, which is anatomically in line with the right atrium when the patient is lying on his or her back (CVP normal value 3–7 mmHg).

Blood pressure

Arterial pressure is usually monitored via an indwelling radial artery catheter or, occasionally, by a femoral artery catheter. The pressure is displayed digitally and in waveform on the bedside monitor.

The radial artery is the most common insertion site. This has many benefits, not least because it is easily observable. As with any invasive line it shares the same complications, although dislodgement and bleeding can result in more rapid haemodynamic instability when compared with a peripheral cannula or even central lines.

Thrombosis is an irritating complication and will prevent the arterial line being beneficial to the patient. It needs to be patent to allow for continuous blood pressure monitoring and blood gas estimations. When occlusion is suspected, manipulation of the catheter may be beneficial, but forceful flushing is not recommended because this may result in asymptomatic thrombus being dislodged. All arterial lines should be connected to a continuous heparinised flush, and display of the waveform on a bedside monitor should provide a good indication of its function. As a result of taking arterial blood gases, the flush circuit is interrupted and infection can result, so strict attention to hygiene is required. Most centres advocate the use of transparent dressings to facilitate observation, and this is usually secured by a pressure dressing. The arterial line is usually clearly marked to avoid accidental injection of substances that could cause arterial spasm and potential necrosis.

Arterial lines could have a detrimental effect on the circulation in the patient's hand. Before insertion the circulation in the patient's hand should have been assessed using Allen's test. In addition, when blood is taken for sampling, the hand should be observed for blanching, which should alert the nurse to deficits in circulation; removal is advocated in these circumstances.

Hypertension is thought to exist in 30–50% (Harlan et al., 1995) of patients after cardiopulmonary bypass. It commonly results from enhanced sympathetic nervous system activity caused by elevated levels of noradrenaline (norepinephrine), renin–angiotensin and vasopressin, which are associated with the use of the extracorporeal circulation. It is an undesirable situation in the postoperative period because it can predispose to bleeding (see Chapter 7), cause suture line disruption and aortic dissection, resulting in an increased oxygen demand by the myocardium, and can depress myocardial performance.

Parameters are commonly set to maintain the systolic blood pressure (e.g. systolic blood pressure 100–140 mmHg). These parameters are usually determined by individual patient differences, and the type of surgery performed. A patient with previous hypertension may require a higher systolic pressure to maintain renal function. After surgery for an aortic root replacement or aortic dissection repair, a patient may require a lower systolic pressure to reduce the pressure on the suture line.

After coronary artery bypass grafting, hypertension could impact on the patency of the grafted vessels. Glyceryl trinitrate (GTN) can assist in controlling hypertension by reducing afterload, but also by maintaining the patency of any grafted vessels. Sodium nitroprusside, another short-acting vasodilator, can also be used. The use of antiplatelet agents, e.g. aspirin, in promoting the patency of vein grafts is well established and some agent is started in all patients unless they are on an anticoagulant for atrial fibrillation. Hypertension or hypotension is avoided by the management of blood volume and drug therapy. The patient with treated hypertension before surgery does not necessarily require the use of anti-hypertensive agents during early convalescence.

Sodium nitroprusside is a vasodilator that has a direct effect on vascular smooth muscle, affecting both arteries and veins, and it effects a reduction in pre-load and afterload. It can be administered only via a continuous intravenous infusion, onset of action occurring after a maximum of 2 minutes, with a shorter half-life. If the infusion is not covered to protect it from light, the liquid can turn into cyanide. The usual response to sodium nitroprusside is a fall in blood pressure by 30–40%, and it should therefore not be administered if the systolic blood pressure is less than 100 mmHg. It is ideally given centrally; peripheral administration may result in a delay in action, particularly in a vasoconstricted patient.

The administration of inotropic drugs increases the force and extent of myocardial fibre shortening, which results in improved emptying of the ventricle with each beat, thereby improving cardiac output. The ideal drug should increase myocardial contractility without affecting heart rate, cause cardiac rhythm disturbances or increase peripheral resistance.

The main drugs used to gain this effect are adrenaline, noradrenaline and dobutamine.

Patients who have continuing hypertension postoperatively may require oral antihypertensives. Once haemodynamic stability is established, and weaning from ventilation has occurred, continuous blood pressure monitoring continues until the arterial line is removed. Even when the arterial line is *in situ*, the accuracy must be checked by re-zeroing the transducer and ensuring that the placement of the transducer is consistent. The frequency of monitoring thereafter can be reduced, the speed of this often being determined by locally devised criteria. Blood pressure should not be recorded after the patient has just mobilised.

Haemodynamic pressure monitoring

Flow directed pulmonary artery catheters were initially introduced by Dr Swan and Dr Ganz and are still referred to as Swan–Ganz catheters. They allow for the measurement of pulmonary artery wedge (PAW) pressure which is an index of left ventricular function. The tip of the catheter has a balloon, which when inflated causes the tip of the catheter to become buoyant. When advanced, the catheter will float in the direction of the blood flow. It can then be passed into the right atrium, through the tricuspid valve into the right ventricle, through the pulmonary valve and into the pulmonary artery, and the tip should lie less than 2 cm from the hilum of the pulmonary artery (Figure 5.5). If advanced further, the catheter will obstruct forward blood flow, which allows left heart pressures to be reflected though the catheter tip. It is indicated when accurate measurements of fluid status, cardiovascular function, and oxygen delivery and consumption are required.

If problems have been encountered during surgery, the pulmonary artery catheter may be positioned when in the operating room, but only after the surgery has been completed to avoid the risks of accidentally suturing part of the catheter during the procedure. Alternatively, this may be positioned in intensive care. For this procedure, the patient must be placed in the Trendelenburg position to allow for identification of the subclavian vein and to reduce the risks of air embolism. Figure 5.6 illustrates the waveforms to be seen on the bedside monitor as the catheter is passed through the heart.

The pressure generated by myocardial contraction and relaxation are reflected through the lumen of the catheter to the transducer, where the pressure is converted to an electrical waveform. For accurate pressure measurement, the transducer must be zeroed and placed at a standard level in relation to the patient position – midchest may suffice as this

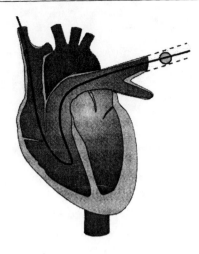

Figure 5.5 Correct placement of a pulmonary artery catheter. Reproduced with permission. From Bloe (1994) Use of a pulmonary artery flotation catheter in a coronary care unit. *British Journal of Nursing* 3: 16.

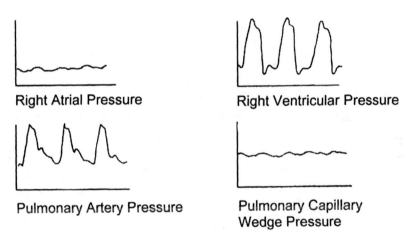

Right Atrial Pressure

Right Ventricular Pressure

Pulmonary Artery Pressure

Pulmonary Capillary Wedge Pressure

Figure 5.6 Waveform changes during pulmonary artery catheter insertion. Reproduced with permission. From Bloe (1994) Use of a pulmonary artery flotation catheter in the coronary care unit. *British Journal of Nursing* 3: 16.

reference level. Accuracy of readings has been shown with a backrest elevation at 30° and 60° (Cline and Gurka 1991), providing that the reference point remains constant (Brandsetter et al., 1998). Measurement in the sitting position is not recommended, and there is inadequate research to justify the use of the lateral position. Therefore, providing that the patient is supine and the point of reference remains constant, there is flexibility around the positioning of the patient.

Zeroing

The transducer must be set at an arbitrarily assigned zero value pressure. This can be done by opening the transducer to room air or atmospheric pressure (760 mmHg at sea level), and assigning that pressure zero value in millimetres of mercury. The pressure module allows the transducer to be zeroed and calibrated, and the pressure waveform to be continuously displayed on an oscilloscope. When changes occur in the waveform configuration, the possible causes need to be considered. While the catheter is *in situ*, the pulmonary artery trace should be apparent unless the catheter is being 'wedged'. A pulmonary artery waveform that becomes flattened is said to be 'damped'. Damped waveforms occur when there is air in the fluid line, when intravenous flow rate decreases and blood stasis occurs, when a fibrin clot is in the catheter tip, or when the catheter adheres to the vessel wall, so flushing the line may restore the waveform.

Problems related to a pulmonary artery catheter

Although there are many risks, they tend to be relatively uncommon and may have a positive link to user experience. The complications may occur in any of three stages: insertion, while indwelling and on removal (complications summarised in Table 5.2).

Flotation of the balloon is achieved through a 2- to 3-ml syringe attached to the balloon lumen. The catheter can become wedged in the pulmonary capillary bed by inflating the balloon or by advancing the catheter into the pulmonary artery, but accidental inflation of the balloon needs to be considered. There may be spontaneous wedging with the balloon deflated as a result of the catheter advancing into a smaller branch of the artery. This may occur as the catheter warms to body temperature, straightens and advances peripherally with the flow of blood, and pulmonary ischaemia occurs in up to 7% of patients. Failure to identify a prolonged wedge trace may lead to pulmonary infarction as a result of an interruption in blood flow. The catheter tip may sometimes float into the right ventricle and the waveform will change. This may predispose to ventricular dysrhythmias and the balloon will not wedge. Alteration of the waveform, not connected to balloon inflation, requires manipulation of the catheter. This is currently predominantly performed by medical staff. If the catheter is to be withdrawn slightly, the balloon should be deflated, and inflated only during advancement of the catheter. The incidence of malpositioning is as high as 25% (Juniper and Gerrard,

Table 5.2 The complications associated with pulmonary artery catheters

Potential complications on insertion and advancement
Vascular damage (venous and arterial)
Haematoma
Infection
Local thrombus
Premature atrial contractions
Premature ventricular contractions
Ventricular fibrillation
Chronic heart block (in patients with existing left bundle-branch block)
Right bundle-branch block

Potential associated complications during indwelling period
Thrombosis
Bacteraemia
Endocarditis
Valve rupture
Pneumothorax
Pulmonary embolism
Pulmonary infarction
Pulmonary artery rupture
Pulmonary infiltrates
Arrhythmia (on injection during output studies)

Potential complications on removal
Inserted preoperatively – accidentally sewn to the wall of the pulmonary artery
Asystolic arrest
Knotting of catheter
Dysrhythmias

1997), and increases the risk of complications. Imaging is therefore important to confirm acceptable positioning of the catheter.

If the balloon is over-inflated, the pulmonary artery may rupture. The artery may also be pierced by an unprotected tip (a deflated balloon) during manipulation. When this occurs, the patient's respiratory status may deteriorate and will require removal of blood from the lungs, usually by bronchoscopy. Occasionally, the balloon itself may rupture and, although this means that a small volume of air is injected into the circulation, it is of little consequence if identified immediately. A ruptured balloon may be suspected if the catheter cannot be wedged and blood is detected in the line. However, if the catheter is left *in situ*, continued attempts to wedge the balloon may result in dangerous levels of air being injected into the patient.

Long-term pulmonary artery catheterisation has been associated with damage to valve cusps as a result of repeated closure of the valves on the line. Removal must never be attempted with the balloon inflated because this will cause severe valve damage. Occasionally, the catheter can become looped or knotted. If this happens, it usually occurs in the right ventricle and will be seen on a radiograph after insertion. Surgery may be required to remove the catheter should kinking occur. As for insertion, during removal the bedside monitor should be continuously observed for dysrhythmias. Baldwin and Heland (2000) suggest that 19% of patients experience cardiac dysrhythmias during removal. These are usually self-terminating but may induce a short period of hypotension. If the introducer sheath also has to be removed, the patients should be placed in the supine or Trendelenburg position to minimise the risk of air embolism.

Catheter care

The presence of any invasive line into a vessel increases the likelihood of infection. Measures to reduce infection are discussed in Chapter 10. The incidence of local and systemic infection increases after the catheter has been *in situ* for 3 days. The catheter should remain *in situ* only as long as is necessary and elective replacement should be considered if continued use is required.

Cardiac output studies

The thermodilution catheter remains a diagnostic device, because the insertion of a catheter alone cannot improve the outcome. Outcome can be affected only by action taken on the results of cardiac output studies, and this action is more frequently becoming a nursing role. Cardiac output is the primary determinant of measuring the ability of the cardiovascular system to deliver oxygen to the body's tissues. Accuracy in obtaining cardiac output readings depends on the delivery of the precise amount of injected volume as programmed into the computer, and a consistent injection rate (<4 seconds for 10 ml). Even with an error-free technique, results have an accuracy of only 10–15%. Cardiac output may be inadequate in tricuspid insufficiency, bidirectional shunts and atrial fibrillation.

Normal cardiac output at rest is considered to be 4–7 l/min, but actual cardiac output is related to body size. The cardiac index is a more realistic guide for evaluating the cardiac output of any individual. The cardiac index is obtained by dividing the cardiac output by the body surface area. This is usually calculated by the computer by entering the patient's height and weight; it is also determined in the preoperative preparation (see Chapter 2). A normal cardiac index is 2.5–4 1/min per m².

Low cardiac output

Low cardiac output is the most critical physiological abnormality in the cardiac surgical patient. A decrease in the pumping effectiveness of the left ventricle results in a decrease in the pressure generated within the ventricle, causing the cardiac output to fall. Venous return to the right side of the heart is a major factor in determining cardiac output. The heart can pump only the volume presented to it, and cardiac output falls if there is inadequate blood volume. Low cardiac output caused by decreased venous return is commonly the result of severe haemorrhage or postoperative dehydration. Intraoperative factors include inadequate myocardial revascularisation, hibernating myocardium, poor myocardial protection, stunned myocardium and reperfusion injury. However, it must be remembered that patients receiving positive pressure mechanical ventilation may have a decreased cardiac output as a result of the absence of the normal drop in intrathoracic pressure on inspiration, a mechanism that normally assists venous return.

The development of a severe low-cardiac output state may lead to secondary system failure, including renal, cerebral and gastrointestinal system failure, and a higher risk of wound infection. Patients with a previously identified poor left ventricle or who present with a low cardiac output state may be given a bolus of calcium intravenously in an attempt to improve myocardial contractility.

High cardiac output

Cardiac output increases with exercise as a result of increased oxygen consumption at a cellular level. Stimulation of the sympathetic nervous system will increase cardiac output by increasing heart rate and the contractile force of the left ventricle.

With the introduction of four-lumen thermodilution catheters and cardiac output computers, it is now a relatively simple procedure to measure cardiac output. When thermodilution is used, the indicator is a cold solution (5% dextrose or 0.9% saline) injected into the right atrium, and the sampling device is a thermistor near the end of the catheter in the pulmonary artery. The thermistor continuously measures the temperature of blood flowing past it. The catheter is connected to the cardiac output computer which determines the cardiac output from the time–temperature curve, which in turn results from the rate of change in temperature of the blood that flows past the thermistor. Debate has arisen as to how cold the injector fluid should be, but there has been no conclusive result. It is vital, however, that the injected fluid is 2°C lower than the body temperature to ensure that there is a temperature gradient.

Systemic vascular resistance (SVR) reflects the resistance to blood flow in the entire systemic circulation. To calculate this, the pressure difference between the proximal (central venous) and distal (mean arterial) ends of the cardiovascular system is divided by cardiac output. The value is multiplied by the conversion factor (79.96) which changes units of mmHg/l per min to dyn/s per cm^3. A decreasing SVR suggests a general vasodilatory reaction. Increasing values are indicative of general vasoconstriction (e.g. cardiogenic/hypovolaemic shock) as a result of compensatory sympathetic nervous system activity in order to maintain blood pressure. The value is clinically useful in determining whether the patient requires vasodilators or vasoconstrictors to improve cardiac function.

It is important to remember that a major determinant of cardiac output is venous return and vascular resistance. If cardiac output is altered, filling pressures and SVR require review to give an indication of the problem and required treatment.

Steps must be taken to eliminate errors because chemical agents may be adjusted in response to the results obtained. Lines should be re-zeroed when the patient is calm and in the supine position. The cardiac rhythm should be observed immediately after the injection, because the sudden bolus of cold solution into the right atrium may precipitate atrial and ventricular dysrhythmias. Three to four consecutive readings should be taken and an average obtained. The cardiac output and cardiac index should always be evaluated in conjunction with other assessed parameters and the clinical status of the patient.

Intra-aortic balloon counterpulsation

Indications

The intra-aortic balloon pump (IABP) is a cardiac assist device designed to increase coronary perfusion and decrease myocardial oxygen consumption (Table 5.3 shows the indications for use). The balloon catheter is usually inserted percutaneously through the femoral artery. It is positioned in the descending thoracic aorta, distal to the left subclavian artery; the tip, as well as the whole length of the balloon, can be identified by radio-opaque markers. Proximal location risks occlusion of the left subclavian or carotid artery, and distal positioning reduces the efficacy of augmentation and risks occlusion of the abdominal vessels. Daily imaging is required because the tip position may vary after repositioning of the patient. It is connected to a console, which shuttles helium in and out of the balloon to inflate and deflate it in cycle with the mechanical cardiac cycle. It increases aortic pressure during diastole to augment coronary perfusion and decreases aortic pressure during systole to lessen the workload on the left ventricle. The balloon is inflated during diastole and deflated during systole. (Figures 5.7 and 5.8 show the positioning of the balloon during diastole and systole.)

The balloon can be triggered by several methods including ECG, pressure, pacing and internal. The ECG is the most common trigger method, and in this mode the balloon deflation occurs on the R wave. In the pressure mode, inflation of the balloon is triggered by the dicrotic notch. In pacing mode, the pacing spike acts as the trigger.

Table 5.3 Summary of the intra-aortic balloon pump

Indications
Refractory ventricular failure
Cardiogenic shock
Unstable refractory angina
Impending infarction
Mechanical complications of myocardial infarction
Ischaemia related to intractable ventricular dysrhythmias
Cardiac support for high-risk surgical patients
Septic shock
Weaning from cardiopulmonary bypass
Intraoperative pulsatile flow generation
Support for failed angioplasty and valvuloplasty

Contraindications
Severe aortic insufficiency
Abdominal or aortic aneurysm
Severe calcific aortic iliac disease or peripheral vascular disease

Adverse effects
Balloon membrane perforation
Limb ischaemia
Bleeding at the insertion site
Infection
Thrombocytopenia
Aortic dissection
Thrombosis

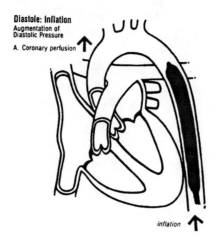

Figure 5.7 The intra-aortic balloon during diastole: augmentation of diastolic pressure increased coronary perfusion. Reproduced with kind permission of Datascope Medical Co. Ltd.

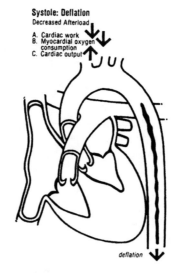

Figure 5.8 The intra-aortic balloon during systole: decreased afterload, reduced cardiac work, reduced myocardial oxygen consumption and increased cardiac output. Reproduced with kind permission of Datascope Medical Co. Ltd.

The frequency with which the balloon inflates can also be manipulated. Most machines have a frequency of 1:1, 1:2 and 1:3. In the ratio 1:1, the balloon inflates with every cardiac cycle and this is used for most patients on initiation and when haemodynamic instability is present. The ratio of 1:1 will be discontinued when the patient either shows improvement and is to be weaned off the balloon pump, or is in rapid atrial fibrillation when the machine has difficulty in identifying the trigger. Altering the ratio to 1:2 reduces the support to the heart by 60%. The 1:3 ratio is predominantly used as a weaning mode. Caution is stressed when reducing augmentation as a weaning method, in that it is difficult to visualise the amount of balloon inflation occurring within the aorta, and the need to ensure that the catheter does not remain immobile or 'flutter' for more than 30 min. Weaning by reducing the ratio is therefore advocated. Table 5.4 suggests the criteria used for weaning off the balloon pump.

The effectiveness of the therapy relies on correct augmentation of the balloon and correct timing. Inflation of the balloon is timed to occur at the dicrotic notch on the arterial pressure tracing. As the balloon inflates, diastolic pressure is augmented, increasing both coronary artery blood flow and myocardial oxygen supply. The balloon must be deflated when the aortic valve opens and the most effective time for this is immediately before the aortic valve opens. Deflation of the balloon decreases the aortic end-diastolic pressure. The optimal timing of deflation is that which gives the greatest drop in aortic end-diastolic pressure (a 5–15 mmHg drop in end-diastolic pressure can be achieved). Correct timing of deflation will also lower peak systolic pressure. The pressure waveform in a patient receiving IAB counterpulsation is shown in Figure 5.9. Incorrect timing,

Table 5.4 Criteria to be used when weaning off intra-aortic balloon counterpulsation

Haemodynamic stability
Cardiac index >2 l/min
PCWP < 22 mmHg
Systolic BP > 90 mmHg
Mean arterial pressure > 70 mmHg
Decreasing inotropic support

Evidence of good coronary perfusion
Absence of life-threatening arrhythmias
Absence of ischaemia on ECG

Evidence of adequate cardiac perfusion
Good peripheral pulses
Adequate urine output
Absence of pulmonary oedema
Improved neurological status (if not sedated)

Balloon needs to be removed if severe vascular insufficiency
Balloon leakage
Deteriorating irreversible condition
PCWP, pulmonary capillary wedge pressure.

i.e. late deflation or early inflation, may counter the beneficial effects of the therapy and increase myocardial oxygen requirements.

During IABP therapy the bedside monitor, in registering blood pressure, identifies the highest and lowest arterial pressures, namely a false systolic (diastolic augmentation) and assisted end-diastolic pressure. A more reliable blood pressure can be obtained from the balloon console, but the mean arterial pressure is a more reliable pressure when estimating the beneficial effects of therapy.

Mean arterial pressure is calculated by subtracting diastolic pressure from systolic pressure, dividing by three and adding this to the systolic pressure. The mathematical mean is not used because systole is sustained for approximately one-third of the cardiac cycle whereas diastole lasts for about two-thirds.

There are several adverse effects associated with the balloon (highlighted in Table 5.3), the risk of which increases with the duration of therapy. Good nursing care and patient observation can result in the early identification of adverse effects, and the appropriate treatment can be initiated.

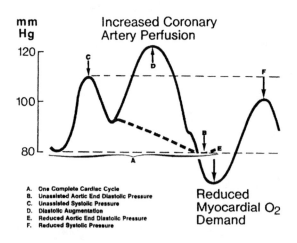

A. One Complete Cardiac Cycle
B. Unassisted Aortic End Diastolic Pressure
C. Unassisted Systolic Pressure
D. Diastolic Augmentation
E. Reduced Aortic End Diastolic Pressure
F. Reduced Systolic Pressure

Figure 5.9 Arterial waveform during therapy by intra-aortic balloon pump (IABP). Reproduced with kind permission of Datascope Medical Co. Ltd.

Balloon membrane perforation

This can occur before, during or after insertion. The main causes of perforation are contact with a sharp instrument, fatigue failure as a result of unusual folding of the balloon membrane during use, and contact with calcified plaque resulting in abrasion of the surface and eventual perforation. When perforation occurs, blood may become visible in the IAB catheter. Other indicators can occur, including IABP leak alarm, dried blood particles or serosanguineous fluid seen in the extracorporeal tubing or catheter extender, or a sudden change in the diastolic augmentation pressure waveform. In the event of a perforation the following action should occur immediately:

- IABP should be stopped and tubing clamped
- remove the IAB catheter within 30 min
- place the patient in the Trendelenburg position
- replace the IAB catheter if the patient condition warrants.

To continue to pump an IAB that has a leak could result in gaseous embolic injury of organs, or a large blood clot may form within the balloon membrane which necessitates surgical removal, even after percutaneous incision. Perforation of a balloon membrane may indicate that the patient's vascular condition may induce abrasion or perforation in subsequent balloon membranes.

Limb ischaemia

Limb ischaemia has been defined as diminished or absent pulses, abnormal temperature, change in colour, pain in the affected limb and gangrene that may require amputation. The description is broad and as a result this complication occurs in 14–45% of patients.

The patient must be consistently observed for any signs of ischaemia both during and for 2 hours after removal. The presence of distal pulses and adequate capillary refill should be assessed before and immediately after balloon insertion, and during the course of therapy. Pulses should be assessed hourly and documented. In addition, the radial pulse in the left arm should be monitored as a result of the risk of the smaller catheters migrating into the left subclavian artery. It may be necessary to locate the pulse using a Doppler monitor if there is any doubt. If a clinically significant decrease of pulse to the affected limb is observed the risk:benefit ratio needs to be reassessed and the removal of the balloon may be necessary based on the clinical judgement of medical staff.

It has been suggested that the development of limb ischaemia may be associated with specific cardiac risk factors, such as peripheral vascular disease, diabetes, age and the smaller vasculature of females. During balloon inflation, there is not total occlusion of the aorta so ischaemic damage to tissue is avoided. It is possible to perform cardiac catheterisation in patients when the balloon pump is in operation, which demonstrates the space occupied by the balloon.

After removal of the IAB, compartment syndrome may occur. In addition to observing the limb for bleeding and pulses, the limb should be assessed for swelling and/or hardness. If this is identified, calf girth measurements should be taken.

Bleeding at the insertion site

Bleeding at the insertion site may be caused by trauma to the artery during insertion of the IAB, excessive catheter movement at the insertion site and excessive anticoagulation. This can be detected from sudden deterioration of haemodynamic stability or by direct observation. Ideally, any bleeding from the insertion site should be detected by observing the groin anteriorly and posteriorly not just during therapy, but also after removal. The risk can be reduced by suturing the catheter in place and ensuring that the patient remains calm and cooperative, although bleeding can be controlled by applying direct pressure. Anticoagulation is required for the duration of therapy and levels of activated partial thromboplastin time (APPT) should be monitored. Many centres advocate stopping the heparin infusion 4 hours before balloon removal to allow clotting levels to return to normal limits.

Thrombocytopenia

This may result from the action of the balloon catheter on platelets (the mechanical action of persistent inflation and deflation that destroys circulating platelets), and may worsen the damage already resulting from the cardiopulmonary bypass. Although it may be suspected by a general ooziness in the patient, a daily platelet count is required for a more accurate detection. Strict monitoring of heparin therapy is required.

Infection

Infection resulting solely from IABP therapy is a rare complication. However, there are occasions where redness, swelling or pruritus at the insertion site may occur. It may be controlled with careful, sterile technique during dressing changes, occlusion dressings and treatment of any patient discomfort. If the insertion site becomes purulent and the patient manifests leucocytolysis or fever, the site should be cultured to determine micro-organism involvement. If indicated, appropriate antibiotic therapy should be initiated along with reassessment of the risks and benefits of continued IABP therapy.

Aortic dissection

This usually occurs during insertion which, where possible, should occur under fluoroscopy to detect such abnormalities, although this is not always possible. Otherwise resection can be detected by symptoms including back pain and/or abdominal pain, a decreased haematocrit and haemodynamic instability.

Thrombus formation

Thrombosis potentially occurs during counterpulsation. The symptoms associated with thrombus formation and treatment will depend on the organ system involved. The risk of thrombus formation can be reduced by ensuring that the catheter is continually flushed with heparinised saline. This should be complimented by bolus flushes, which are advocated at regular intervals, but it is important that the balloon is not operational during the flush to minimise the risk of flush only being shunted around the coronary arteries during balloon inflation, causing myocardial ischaemia.

A thrombus can form quickly if the balloon becomes immobile. Immobility of the balloon catheter may occur if there is a mechanical fault with the balloon, or at the loss of the patient trigger. The main action is to restart the pumping action but it is important that the intra-aortic balloon is not left immobile in the patient for more than 30 min.

On removal

Pressure should be applied below the puncture site during IAB removal. Free proximal bleeding is allowed for a few seconds, and then pressure is applied above the puncture site, allowing a few seconds of back bleeding. Haemostasis is established by applying pressure to the puncture site for approximately 30 min. The limb distal to the insertion site should be observed for adequate perfusion and the pressure adjusted accordingly.

References

Baldwin I, Heland M (2000) Incidence of cardiac dysrhythmias in patients during pulmonary artery catheter removal after cardiac surgery. *Heart Lung* **29**: 155–60.

Brandsetter R, Grant E, Estilo M, Hahim F, Singh F, Gitter B (1998) Swan–Ganz catheter: Misconceptions, pitfalls and incomplete user knowledge, an identified trilogy in need of correction. *Heart Lung* **27**: 218–22.

Cline J, Gurka A (1991) Effect of backrest position of pulmonary artery pressure and cardiac output measurements in critically ill patients. *Crit Care Nurse* **18**: 283–9.

Gray P, Sullivan G, Ostryzniuk P, McEwen TA (1992) Value of post procedural chest radiographs in the adult intensive care unit. *Crit Care Med* **20**: 1513–16.

Harlan BJ, Starr A, Harwin RM (1995) *Illustrated Handbook of Cardiac Surgery*, Chap. 5. London: Springer, p. 55.

Jackson C (1998) Bedside cardiac monitoring. *Crit Care Nurse* **18**(3): 82–5.

Johnson K (2000) Use of telephone follow-up for post cardiac surgery patients. *Intensive Crit Care Nursing* **16**: 144–50.

Johnson L, Brown G, Alligood M (1993) Complications of epicardial pacing wire removal. *J Cardiovasc Nursing* **7**: 133.

Juniper MC, Gerrard CS (1997) The chest x-ray in intensive care. *Care of the Critically Ill* **13**: 198–200.

Kolvekar S, D'Souza, Akhatar P (1997) Role of atrial ischaemia in the development of atrial fibrillation following coronary artery bypass surgery. *Eur J Cardiothorac Surg* **11**: 70–5.

CHAPTER 6

Maintaining the patient's neurological welfare

Neurological impairment

With the increasing average age of patients undergoing cardiac surgery, and the increasing proportion of complex procedures, there has been a slight increase in neurological complications over the last decade. Some postoperative neurological deficits are minor, and their treatment is of short duration requiring little more than ordinary care and resolving in 2 to 3 days. More severe or persistent defects require a more exhaustive neurological evaluation.

The frequency of neurological injury after cardiac surgery is variable. Cerebrovascular accident (CVA) is the most serious neurological complication, occurring in 0.4–5.4% of patients after coronary artery bypass grafts (CABGs) (Bernat, 1997). Postoperative CVA is defined as a new neurological deficit which lasts at least 24 hours and occurs within 24 hours of surgery (Shaw et al., 1987). This complication is thought to prolong hospital stay by 9 days (Naughton et al., 1999). The risk of postoperative neurological injury in cardiac surgical patients is thought to be related to three factors:

1. patient's preoperative condition
2. equipment/technique used intraoperatively (atherosclerotic debris from the ascending aorta or air embolism from the cardiopulmonary bypass)
3. management of the patient immediately after surgery.

Patients generally undergo surgery with a hope of an improved quality of life. Postoperative CVA is a devastating complication that will further compromise a patient's quality of life.

Preoperative condition

A number of preoperative conditions contribute to the potential for CVA (Table 6.1). Some of these factors – obesity, diet and alcohol consumption – can be modified. Advanced age is probably the greatest preoperative risk factor. The prevalence for stroke rises dramatically with age. The risk of stroke is 0.9% for patients aged under 65 years old and 8.9% for patients over 75 years old (Tuman et al., 1992).

Table 6.1 Preoperative risk factors predisposing to cerebrovascular accident (CVA)

Factor	Reason
Advanced age	Atherosclerosis more likely to be present
Race	Black men have a higher prevalence of hypertension and cerebrovascular accidents
Hypertension	Increased cerebral blood flow and pressure
Obesity	Increased lipid levels
Diabetes mellitus	Elevated glucose levels and vascular plaque
Alcohol consumption	Increased blood viscosity
Diet	Elevated levels of lipids and triglycerides
Coronary artery disease	Formation of plaque that may embolise
Atrial rhythm disorders	Thrombi that may cause emboli
Carotid artery occlusion	Decreased cerebral perfusion
Myocardial infarction	Decreased cerebral perfusion
Previous cardiac surgery	Low-flow state/atherosclerosis

Postoperative considerations

The neurological objective of cardiac surgery is to ensure adequate cerebral blood flow and to prevent emboli originating in the heart from travelling to the brain. The cardiopulmonary bypass, in particular, exposes the central nervous system to a variety of potential effects. These conditions can be mechanical, temperature related, haemodynamic, metabolic or pharmacological. The reduction of cerebral perfusion pressure combined with atherosclerotic disease significantly increases the risk for CVA.

Severe aortic atheroma creates a challenge for cardiac surgeons. The ascending aorta must be cross-clamped to allow for cannulation, but the clamping and later release of clamps allow an atheroma to mobilise and lodge in the cerebral circulation.

The most common form of stroke in the perioperative period appears to have an embolic rather than haemodynamic origin and is usually due to disturbances in atrial rhythm (Harrison, 1995). Most strokes occur postoperatively when systolic blood pressure is adequate, rather than intraoperatively when blood pressure is low (Lindsey, 1998). Postoperatively, a fine balance is needed to control blood pressure, bleeding and oxygenation in order to maintain adequate perfusion of the brain. Inadequate perfusion caused by hypotension or significant bleeding can cause an ischaemic episode, whereas a hypertensive episode can cause increased cerebral flow with the potential for rupture of a blood vessel.

Hypothermia in the initial stage of a patient's recovery can result in sluggish reaction of thought processes, together with a loss of coordination, but these may also be masked by anaesthesia, and it can make immediate postoperative neurological examination difficult. However, after an hour of discontinuing sedation, the patient should have recovered sufficiently to allow for a full neurological assessment and, if any deficits are observed at that time, which are additional to the preoperative condition, the possibility of a neurological insult should be questioned.

Manifestations of a stroke may include any of the following: motor, speech or language deficits, and/or unilateral neglect. Frequent neurological assessments are essential for determining whether the patient's condition is improving, remaining the same or deteriorating. It is the possibility of deterioration that causes most concern. Neurological checks are performed hourly until the patient awakens from anaesthesia, and then the interval between assessments is 2- to 4-hourly depending on the patient's individual condition. Eye opening, obeying commands, moving all four extremities with equal strength and the occurrence of seizure activity should be assessed. Any deficits recognised at this time are crucial, and the information must be communicated to the surgeon.

The Glasgow Coma Scale (GCS) is the method most commonly used to assess a patient's level of consciousness and this is an integral component of neurological examination in a potentially neurologically impaired patient. The GCS is a clinical scale designed to assess the depth of impaired consciousness and coma, and was developed in the 1970s to avoid ambiguities and misunderstandings in the assessment of conscious level. It measures three aspects of a patient's behaviour: eye opening, verbal response and motor response.

Eye opening

A patient is deemed to have spontaneous eye opening if his or her eyes are open without any stimulation on the nurse's behalf. It is possible to make the observation from the foot of the bed without a word being spoken or the patient disturbed. Eye opening is then assessed in response to speech. The patient should be approached in a normal voice (without additional touching or shouting). If this is insufficient to gain a response, greater verbal stimulus is required, and the voice should be raised. Any words or commands may be used, but the patient's hearing should be considered at this point of the assessment.

If no response is achieved, a painful stimulus must be used. In the first instance this involves simply touching the patient's hand or shoulder and shaking him or her. If a deeper stimulus is required, a peripheral pain stimulus should be used. The patient's finger is placed between the nurse's thumb and a 2-ml syringe or pen. Pressure is gradually increased over a matter of seconds until the best response is seen. Any finger can be used, but the third and fourth are thought to be the most sensitive digits. Peripheral pain is used rather than central pain, because the latter will often cause eye closure by inducing a grimacing effect. No response will be recorded when the nurse is sure that sufficient stimuli have been used and the eyes have still not opened.

Verbal response

Eye opening is closely related to being awake and alert. Orientation is the recognition of one's position in relation to time and space. A person who is orientated knows who he is, where he is and when it is. If these three questions are answered correctly he can be classified as orientated, even if other elements of the conversation are confused. If one or more of the questions are incorrectly answered, the patient can be classified as confused. A patient may vary in the degree of disorientation at any given time.

Differentiating between confused conversation and inappropriate words may be difficult. With inappropriate words conversation exchange is absent, there is a tendency to use words more than sentences and replies are usually obtained by physical stimulation. Incomprehensible sounds should be noted when a noise is made but no understandable words can be determined either spontaneously or as a result of stimulus. Best verbal response assesses two elements of cerebral functioning. It examines the comprehension and transmission of sensory input, verbal or physical, and it reflects the ability to articulate or express a reply. It is obvious that some patients are unable to be fairly assessed in this category as a result of injury or the presence of an endotracheal (ET) tube, which is likely immediately after cardiac surgery. In this instances a 'T' should be recorded.

Motor response

The best motor response is being able to obey simple commands convincingly. 'Open your eyes' should be avoided because it could be a reflex, and ideally two different commands should be given, or one should be repeated twice. When a patient does not obey commands, painful stimulus should be applied, and any localised response viewed. The purpose of applying pain is to make the patient suffer momentarily without leaving any residual effects. This can be achieved by the trapezius pinch (pinching the muscle between the shoulders) or supraorbital ridge pressure. Sternal rubbing on a sternum that has recently been operated on is not recommended.

If the patient does not obey commands, or localise to pain, a peripheral pain stimulus must be applied. The upper limbs should be assessed and the best response of either arm recorded. The lower limbs cannot be reliably used. Normal flexion is the response expected on touching a live hot plate. It is a combination of movements involving flexion at the elbow, abduction of the upper arm and extension of the wrist, and it is generally rapid. Extension is obviously abnormal and appears as a straightening of the elbow joint with abduction and internal rotation of the limb. It may be accompanied by wrist flexion. No response may occur as a result of disease or trauma, or from drugs such as paralysing agents, and this should be considered on initial return from the operating room. After a stroke, patients demonstrate a profound weakness on the opposite side that is characterised by a decrease or absence of normal muscle tone, immediate loss of fine manipulative skills and a tendency of the affected limbs to move as a whole. Motor testing of extremities can help to determine whether there is a new deficit, weakness or paralysis. A high percentage of stroke patients have denial of illness and a neglect of half of their body and/or environment.

Pupil response

Normal pupils are round and equal with an average size of 2–5 mm. On assessment, the pupils should initially be observed simultaneously to determine size and quality, before checking the reaction to light. Reaction to light may occasionally be sluggish as a result of the anaesthetic, and the size of the pupil may also be influenced by medication, e.g. atropine used to correct a bradycardia may result in dilated pupils, whereas morphine may contribute to pin-point pupils.

The limb strength is measured in response to a command. The patient should be asked to push and pull against the nurse and then recorded as having normal power, a mild weakness or a severe weakness. The assessment of the legs is more subjective. The assessment of the limbs reflects the functioning of each cerebral hemisphere.

Focal central nervous system deficits of varying severity can continue up to discharge, but less than 33% of patients with a definite stroke continue to have any major functional disability at discharge (Sotaniemi, 1995). Slight-to-moderate focal motor deficits seem to resolve within a few weeks. However, those who sustain a major disability persisting to discharge tend to have a long-term prognosis that is identical to those of patients with stroke in general.

Sedation

Most ventilated patients, especially those with a cuffed oral ET tube will require some form of sedation/analgesia at least initially, because it decreases restlessness while also increasing ventilation compliance. By reducing tachycardia and hypertension, factors known to increase myocardial oxygen demand, and by reducing the incidence of arrhythmias, its use facilitates a more stable cardiovascular system. It is important to be able to assess the conscious state of these patients, and obtain an optimum level of sedation/analgesia. An ideal level is suggested to be when the patient is receiving the minimum necessary dosage of analgesia and sedative, but is tolerant and unstressed for the ventilator.

Sedation should be used in conjunction with a sedation scoring system (Table 6.2). The aims of this scoring system are to enable staff to achieve a calm, comfortable patient using the minimum dose of drug necessary and to avoid under- or over-sedation (see Table 6.3 for the effect of over- or under-sedation). Use of the GCS to assess the level of sedation is not valid because it serves to assess neurological function rather than patient comfort. Similarly, a pain assessment scale reviews patient's pain, which accounts for only a part of patient comfort (Saggs, 1998). When sedation is in use, patients should be assessed hourly against a scale and, in addition, neurological assessment should occur at least once every 24 hours. Sedation must be kept to a minimum to avoid complications of prolonged ventilation by preventing the patient from fully awakening and cooperating.

Although small bolus doses may be required for certain procedures, e.g. physiotherapy, sedation is best provided by a continuous infusion to achieve a steady-state control with minimum side effects. Sedation is

Table 6.2 A sedation scoring system – an adaptation of Ramsay's Sedation Score

Score	Characteristics
1	Unmanageable, agitated, disorientated: at this level the patient is showing signs of discomfort, hypertension, tachycardia, failure to synchronise with the ventilator, hypoxia, hypercapnia, and the risk of displacing invasive lines, tubes, etc.
2	Awake: at this level the patient is awake and orientated, requiring minimal or no sedation. They should be self-ventilating via either a mask or endotracheal tube. This level should be achieved before extubation
3	Roused by voice or touch: the patient responds to speech or touch by either squeezing the nurse's hand or blinking. The patient may require bolus sedation, as well as background sedation cover before handling during nursing/medical procedures or physiotherapy
4	Roused by voice or touch: the patient responds to speech or touch by either squeezing the nurse's hand or blinking. The patient does not require bolus sedation and tolerates handling and procedures well.
5	Sluggish level: the patient shows no sign of response to any form of stimulation
6	Flat level: the patient shows no sign of response to any form of stimulation

Sedation levels 3 and 4 are ideal, allowing the patient to tolerate treatments, general nursing care, physiotherapy and suction, without compromising their ventilation or cardiovascular state
Sedation levels 5 and 6 are acceptable only in critically ill unstable patients where heavy sedation is desirable
From Ramsay et al. (1974).

Table 6.3 Risks associated with over- or under-sedation

Risks of under-sedation	Risks of over-sedation
Discomfort	Coma
Pain	Respiratory depression
Hypertension	Hypotension/haemodynamic disturbances
Tachycardia	Bradycardia
Failure of the ventilator to synchronise	Increased protein breakdown
with the patient – causing hypoxia and	Gastrointestinal stasis
hypercapnia	Malabsorption of enteral nutrition
Agitation	Renal failure
Displacement of tubes/catheter/	Immunosuppression
invasive lines	

usually achieved by the administration of a combination of drugs, e.g. analgesia with a sedative. Current practice is to use drug combinations to achieve these effects, with opioids and benzodiazepines being a frequently used pairing. Midazolam and propofol are available as hypnotics for short-term sedation during the postoperative period.

Propofol is a useful sedative, allowing early tracheal extubation, and was licensed for use on patients receiving mechanical ventilation in 1993. It provides good quality titratable sedation and, on discontinuing, an infusion has a rapid and predictable wake-up time. The haemodynamic effects of propofol – moderate vasodilatation, an absence of tachycardia and maintained cardiac output – are all desirable qualities for patients after cardiac surgery. As a result of the potential for patients to be weaned from a ventilator within a few hours, the use of a long-acting sedative has decreased in favour of short-acting agents with a predictable wake-up time.

Prolonged use of propofol may turn urine a greenish colour, particularly as a result of inactive phenol metabolism, and clearance of propofol is unaffected by renal impairment, which suggests that it remains unaffected by renal replacement therapy, e.g. continuous venous haemofiltration. At high infusion rates, it has the potential for reducing the efficiency of the filter used in renal replacement therapy as a result of its lipid formation. Despite its emulsified appearance propofol does not cause unphysiologically high triglyceride levels, unless parental fats are coadministered.

The sedative infusion rates of propofol are generally between 0.5 and 4 mg/kg per h, and the target blood concentration for sedation is 1–2 µg/ml. Doses can be increased every 5–10 minutes until sedation is achieved. Patients wake up when blood concentrations decrease to 1 µg/ml. When an infusion is discontinued, propofol blood concentrations decrease by 50% in 10 min, and most patients wake up between 5 and 15 min after the infusion is discontinued (Sherry, 1997). Bolus dosing should be avoided because it produces high peaks and low troughs.

Propofol has the potential to cause myocardial depression just like other anaesthetic agents, but this usually occurs with boluses on induction, so plasma expanders should be employed to counter any effects. It has no analgesic properties, but when given at a dosage of 5 µg/kg per min, it has amnesic properties (Harvey, 1996).

Nursing considerations with the administration of propofol

Intravenous access

Propofol can irritate peripheral veins, so it must be given through a central or large peripheral intravenous catheter (Covington, 1998). An infusion device is required to titrate the dose to fit the patient's response and level of sedation. The likelihood of infection can be minimised if the intravenous tubing is changed every 24 hours.

Monitoring

Lipid levels should be monitored in patients receiving infusions that continue longer than 72 hours (Lowrey et al., 1996), because continued infusion can result in marked elevation of lipids. Special consideration should be given to lipids if the patient is concurrently receiving total parental nutrition. Triglyceride levels greater than 5.6 mmol/l may require discontinuation of propofol and use of another sedative agent (Covington, 1998).

Pain

It is a natural assumption that a patient undergoing cardiac surgery, which involves the splitting of the sternum or separation of the ribs, will be accompanied by a certain degree of pain; this is confirmed by the routine administration of analgesia during anaesthesia. Postoperative pain is, however, a multi-dimensional phenomenon. Pain may be experienced as a result of surgical incisions, intraoperative manipulation and dissection, acute myocardial ischaemia and dissecting aortic aneurysm, but it may be the result of other iatrogenic factors, including invasive monitoring, and ET tubes, nasogastric tubes, chest drains and urinary catheters.

Postoperative pain after elective cardiac surgery can be defined as iatrogenic. It is acute, of relatively short duration and usually well localised. It is related to the type and length of incision as well as to the degree of surgical trauma. Patients suggest that the wound is the most common site of postoperative pain and report increased pain when the wound site is touched. Incisions are inevitably complicated by the division of small peripheral nerves as well as by a variable amount of tissue trauma. The inflammation that follows is accompanied by a local decrease in the magnitude of stimuli required to elicit pain (primary hyperalgesia).

The complexity of pain is heightened during the immediate postoperative period by the physiological transition that follows cardiac surgery. Combined with the psychological implications of surgery, the physiological transition and treatment interventions at this time complicate the assessment of pain.

Literature surrounding the realm of pain describes it as the result of two factors – 'sensory' and 'reactive' – where 'sensory' describes its type and intensity and 'reactive' refers to the meaning attached to the pain. Individuals identify and give meaning to their pain using environmental, experiential, cultural and pathological factors to influence this meaning. Impending cardiac surgery may be viewed as a positive or negative experience. For some patients, it represents an opportunity to return to a lifestyle they led before their illness; others view the heart as the centre of emotion and the key of life, seeing surgery as a great threat. In addition, hospitalisation may evoke a negative, psychological reaction because the individual may focus on separation from family, isolation, loss of independence and helplessness. The degree of negative response is thought to correlate closely with subsequent pain perception. Ultimately, the provision of adequate pain relief depends more on the patient's perception of pain than on the precise clinical picture or diagnosis. Ignorance of the psychological impact of a pain experience may result in the persistence of a poor recovery and an increased length of stay.

On a patient's initial return from the operating room, when direct communication with the patient is difficult, the nurse has to pre-empt the degree of pain experienced. Postoperative alterations in cardiac function may necessitate the use of vasoactive medication and possibly support devices in order to maintain cardiac output. The persistence of low cardiac output requires the use of inotropic drugs. Their effects produce various combinations of action on the heart rate. In the immediate postoperative period, vasodilators such as glyceryl trinitrate (GTN) are used to achieve controlled dilatation of the vascular bed, with subsequent control of hypertension through a decrease in afterload. Control over cardiovascular status masks normal objective physiological signs of the pain response highlighted in Table 6.4. More frequently, an analgesic agent may be commenced intravenously to dissipate the onset and degree of pain.

The control of incisional pain has been achieved primarily by the use of medication, with opioids being the preferred option. One problem frequently encountered in the postoperative period is inadequate analgesia. It primarily inhibits mobilisation and promotes shallow breathing because of pain. Bernat (1997) states that the 'practical endpoint of analgesia is not the total abolition of pain but the provision of an acceptable degree of comfort permitting deep breathing, coughing and movement with the minimum possible accompanying side effects'. This balance can be difficult to achieve, but nurses are in the ideal position to influence the patient's pain management, through assessment and recording of a patient's pain, psychological preparation, support and reassurance.

Table 6.4 Physiological changes in acute pain

Thoracic pain causes reduction in:
Tidal volume
Vital capacity
Functional residual capacity
Alveolar ventilation
Atelectasis
Sputum retention and infection

Sympathetic over-activity causes:
Tachycardia
Hypertension
Increased systemic vascular resistance
Increased myocardial oxygen consumption

Anxiety that lowers the pain threshold and skeletal muscle spasm causing:
An increase in the amount of pain
Reduced gastric mobility

Hormonal changes causing:
Electrolyte abnormalities
Hyperglycaemia

Some of the responsibility for optimising pain control lies with the patient, but the overall effects of cardiopulmonary bypass include temporary loss of concentration, memory defects and confusion, and disorientation may make rational thought and responsible decisions virtually impossible at this time. Although medical staff prescribe analgesics, much of the responsibility for patient comfort rests with the nurse. Many patients are reluctant to report postoperative pain, and a lack of a pained expression does not necessarily indicate a lack of pain. Many people believe that admission of, or complaints about, pain are a sign of weakness and an inability to cope with the inevitable consequences of surgery. Nurses have been criticised for having a passive role in the management of postoperative pain. They may play down the intensity of a patient's pain as a result of frustration towards the inadequacy of a medical prescription. Analgesia should not be withheld with the aim of speeding up the weaning of ventilation and extubation. The patient requires analgesia after surgery to be comfortable enough to cooperate and breathe effectively.

Current pharmacological techniques of pain management include a multitude of treatments. The combination usually advocated is opioid analgesia, non-opioid analgesia and non-steroidal anti-inflammatory drugs. Administration of analgesia by the intravenous route allows for instant titration. Some centres favour self-administered analgesia, but the fast recovery now witnessed in most of these patients does not make this standard practice. In the immediate postoperative period analgesics may be kept to a minimum for patients requiring short-term ventilation for fear of prolonging ET intubation through respiratory depression. Patients requiring longer-term ventilation are more likely to receive larger doses of analgesics.

Opioids

After cardiac surgery sedation is usually supplemented by opioid analgesia. Opioids can cause respiratory depression. Acting on the brain-stem respiratory centres, they reduce responsiveness to increases in carbon dioxide tension. Therapeutic doses depress all phases of respiratory activity, but rarely to any significant extent, and Porter (1991) suggests that it occurs in less than 1% of patients. Any depression is reversible with the use of parental naloxone hydrochloride, and it should be remembered that pain itself interferes with respiratory function.

Morphine appears to be the opioid of choice and the mainstay of analgesia in the immediate postoperative period. Its precise mechanism is unknown, but morphine alters the perception of pain at the spinal cord with resultant analgesic effect. Its use after cardiac surgery is wholly appropriate despite varied side effects. While reducing myocardial oxygen consumption and workload, it has little effect on heart rate or cardiac output. Argument surrounds the administration of an opioid by continuous infusion and intravenous bolus injection, and there appears to be little difference between the two in analgesic effect. However, as intravenous bolus techniques result in plasma concentration peaks and valleys, and subsequent alterations in haemodynamic stability, the value of continuous intravenous therapy emerges. Continuous intravenous opioid infusions minimise haemodynamic changes, while also providing a means of ongoing analgesia.

The dosage is 2.5–7.5 mg/h by slow intravenous infusion if the patient is experiencing acute pain, but there is no maximum dosage if the patient is in severe pain. There may be a delay in commencing a morphine infusion as a result of the possibility that it may adversely affect a neurological assessment and delay the weaning process. This is a dubious argument because control of pain is always enhanced by preventing the experience.

However, in the presence of renal failure a differing opioid should be used, i.e. alfentanil.

Alfentanil is a potent, short-acting opioid analgesic, with a very rapid onset of action. It has no sedative properties so it should have an accompanying hypnotic or sedative agent. The infusions should be run separately to enable individual titration. Alfentanil is the agent of choice in renal failure because its metabolites are inactive, although the patient may require a reduced dose.

The recommended infusion rate for the mechanically ventilated patient is 2 mg/h. More rapid control may initially be gained by using a loading dose of 5 mg over 10 min. The dose required should be individually determined and reassessed. The dose is generally 0.5–10 mg alfentanil/h. The maximum recommended duration of treatment with alfentanil infusion is 4 days. As with morphine, effects can be reversed with naloxone (Narcan).

Patient-controlled analgesia has been advocated for use in pain management after CABGs. It has proven benefits with alert, orientated and cooperative patients, but its use in the immediate postoperative period may be impractical.

In the early postoperative period the use of an opioid analgesic in combination with a non-opioid analgesic proves more effective than use of opioids alone. Non-opioid analgesics are most effective in the treatment of mild-to-moderate pain of non-visceral origin. However, they need to be used correctly (particularly paracetamol).

Epidural or spinal anaesthesia in cardiac patients is controversial. Among the suggested benefits are better management of pain and earlier mobilisation, but this benefit has to be balanced against risks of spinal haematoma, which could result in death or neurological dysfunction. Patients who have undergone complete heparinisation (necessary for cardiopulmonary bypass) are more susceptible to this complication.

Non-opioid analgesia

Compound analgesic preparations such as co-dydramol and co-proxamol must be regarded with caution. They are used frequently in pain management, but their opioid content may cause significant side effects without any apparent increase in analgesic effect. In addition, they cause constipation, the effects being enhanced in less mobile patients, and it may interact with warfarin particularly when they are taken haphazardly 'as required'.

Non-steroidal anti-inflammatory drugs

The value of non-steroidal anti-inflammatory drugs (NSAIDs) is well documented. NSAIDs inhibit prostaglandin synthesis, modifying the inflammatory response. However, by virtue of their effect on prostaglandin synthesis, NSAIDs can affect renal function adversely. They should be introduced cautiously after cardiac surgery, when acute alterations in renal function frequently occur after cardiopulmonary bypass. NSAIDs also inhibit platelet aggregation, with resultant alterations in haemostasis. These side-effects are generally limited by short-term use of drugs, but their significance cannot be ignored. Before commencing NSAIDs, biochemistry screening should be checked and abnormally high urea and creatinine levels should deter the use of this medication.

A favoured route for NSAIDs is rectal administration, and administration by the blunt end first is thought to aid retention (Addison and Lavender, 2000). When administered rectally, patients should be encouraged to have their bowels open first. The medication starts to take effect after 45 min, but takes up to 6 hours to dissolve fully. NSAIDs should be used cautiously in patients with asthma, in whom the drugs may precipitate severe acute bronchospasm, especially in patients with a history of aspirin intolerance. NSAIDs can impair blood pressure control in hypertensive patients treated with β blockers, angiotensin-converting enzyme (ACE) inhibitors and diuretics.

In addition to administering prescribed analgesics, further practical steps can be taken to maintain a patient's comfort. These include helping patients find a comfortable resting position and encouraging them to support their sternal wound during activities that strain the wound (coughing), and ensuring that analgesia is given at an appropriate time, e.g. before physiotherapy, for removal of chest drains and first thing in the morning when the patient feels stiff from lying in bed.

Postpericardiotomy syndrome is a common complication after cardiac surgery. Diagnosis is based on the presence of at least two of the following: fever, anterior chest pain and friction rub. The effective drug in the relief of this complication is ibuprofen or indomethacin (Horneffer et al., 1990).

Chest wall discomfort is a common complaint among women and for some it remains a characteristic after 18 months. As a result of the sex, it is thought to be an anatomical relationship, the result of tissue and nerve disruption after dissection of the internal mammary artery from the chest wall.

References

Addison R, Lavender R (2000) How to administer enema and suppositories. *Nursing Times* **96**(6): NTPlus Continence 3–4.

Bernat J (1997) Smoothing the CABG patient's road to recovery. *Am J Nursing* **97**(2): 23–7.

Covington H (1998) Use of propofol for sedation in the ICU. *Crit Care Nurse* **18**(4): 34–39.

Harrison MJ (1995) Neurologic complications of coronary artery bypass grafting: diffuse or focal ischaemia? *Ann Thorac Surg* **59**: 1356–8.

Harvey MA (1996) Managing agitation in critically ill patients. *Am J Crit Care* **5**: 7–18.

Horneffer P, Miller R, Pearson TA et al. (1990) The effective treatment of post pericardiotomy syndrome after cardiac operations. A randomised placebo trial. *J Thorac Cardiovasc Surg* **100**: 292–6.

Lindsey M (1998) Frequency of CVA after cardiac surgery. *Crit Care Nurse* **18**(5): 19–25.

Lowrey TS, Dunlap AW, Brown RO, Dickerson RA, Rudsk KA (1996) Pharmacologic influence on nutrition support therapy: use of propofol in a patient receiving combined enteral and parental nutrition support. *Nutr Clin Pract* **11**: 147–9.

Naughton C, Prowroznyk A, Feneck R (1999) Reason for prolonged hospital stays following heart surgery. *Br J Nursing* **8**: 1085–94.

Porter G (1991) Patient controlled analgesia – an anaesthetist's view. *Br J Theatre Nursing* **1**(5): 13–14.

Ramsay M, Savage T, Simpson B et al. (1974) Controlled sedation with alphaxolone–alphadolone. *BMJ* **II**: 656–9.

Saggs P (1998) Sedation scoring in a general ICU – comparative trial of 2 assessment tools in clinical practice. *Nursing Crit Care* **3**(6): 289–365.

Shaw PJ, Bates D, Cartlidge NE et al (1987) Neurologic and neuropsychological morbidity following major surgery: comparison of coronary artery bypass and peripheral vascular surgery. *Stroke* **18**: 700–7.

Sherry KM (1997) The use of propofol for ICU sedation in patients following cardiac surgery. *Br J Intensive Care* **7**(3): 94.

Sotaniemi K (1995) Longterm neurologic outcome after cardiac operation. *Ann Thorac Surg* **59**: 1336–9.

Tuman K, McCarthy R, Najafi H et al. (1992) Differential effect of advanced age: neurologic and cardiac risks of coronary artery operation. *J Thorac Cardiovasc Surg* **104**: 1510–17.

CHAPTER 7

Caring for a patient's nutritional needs

It is now well documented that patients in hospital are prone to malnutrition and the nutritional status of patients is becoming an important consideration even in relatively short-stay patients. The nutritional status of the patient is initially assessed on admission and a variety of scales have been devised. The body mass index provides an indication of obesity based on the patient's height and weight and, in addition, can prompt a weight-reducing diet, but is of less concern with patients who are deemed underweight. As a result of a preoccupation with improving a patient's cardiovascular status, nutritional needs are frequently given minimal attention for most patients.

Patients return from the operating room having been fasted for a minimum of 3 hours preoperatively. This means that, by the time they return from the operating room, the patient has had no oral intake for approximately 7 hours. This in itself can cause the patient discomfort, but the lack of oral hydration combined with medication received during the anaesthetic can make the patient's oral cavity exceeding dry.

While patients remain ventilated, they will still be nil by mouth, and they may or may not have a nasogastric tube in place, depending on the operation performed and the surgeon's preference. The presence of an endotracheal (ET) tube and mechanical ventilation exacerbates a dry mouth, and oral care is of paramount importance. In addition, the bacteria found in the mouth can colonise in the respiratory tract within 24 hours, and good oral hygiene can prevent the potential complication of a chest infection.

Oral care

Oral care is an important part of total patient care. Its major purpose is the maintenance of a functional and comfortable oral cavity, the enhancement of self-esteem, and the reduction of both bacterial activity in the mouth and local and systemic infection. Ventilated patients are generally unable to attend to their own oral hygiene and therefore depend on the nurse to attend to it for them. When the patient is nil by mouth, or drinks less, saliva production is reduced and the cleanliness effect of saliva on the tongue and mucous membrane is lost. Any interruption in saliva production, as a result of dehydration or drug therapy, can lead to infection of the salivary glands by the oral flora.

Diseases of the oral cavity, such as periodontal disease, are recognised risk factors for heart disease. The presence of food is not necessary for the formation of plaque, and it continues to form in the mouth of those who are receiving nil by mouth. Dental plaque is the primary cause of the two major dental diseases: dental decay (caries) and periodontal (gum) disease. Dry mouth (xerostomia) can arise from 400 commonly used drugs, mouth breathing, oxygen therapy, poor appetite, anxiety, general debility and depression.

The toothbrush is the most commonly used tool in the Western World for the maintenance of oral health. This is based on strong evidence to support the toothbrush as the most effective method in the control of dental plaque and its associated complications. Other tools and various solutions used by nurses for mouth care are of unproven value and may be detrimental. They do not add to patient comfort, because they do not remove plaque effectively. Commonly employed treatments include:

- lubrication swabs
- mouth rinses
- sipping water
- swabbing with crushed ice
- saliva substitutes.

Hydration

On return from the operating room, initially the patient will remain nil by mouth until extubation occurs and, once adequate respiratory status has been confirmed by clinical assessment and arterial blood gases, oral fluids may commence. However, if a paralytic ileus is suspected, as a result of surgery (e.g. use of a gastroepiploic artery in bypass grafts), the patient will remain nil by mouth with a nasogastric tube *in situ* until normal bowel sounds have occurred.

During the period of nil by mouth, which is relatively short for most patients, hydration is maintained by an intravenous infusion of crystalloid, usually 5% dextrose. To prevent overhydration and potential pulmonary oedema, the rate of infusion is calculated on an hourly basis, and consideration is given to the amount of fluid administered from other infusions. Hourly fluids are therefore usually calculated to be 1 ml/kg body weight, e.g. a patient of 75 kg will receive an hourly replacement of 75 ml. This replacement fluid also allows some electrolytes to be administered, particularly calcium, which improves myocardial contractility, and potassium. Potassium supplements may be required hourly in light of an expected large diuresis. Maintaining a potassium level between 4.0 and 5.0 mmol/l is an important nursing function. This is initially achieved by intravenous potassium supplements, but hypokalaemia should not always necessitate intravenous correction and oral potassium supplements such as Sando-K can be given. The patients should also be encouraged to eat foods known to have a high potassium content such as oranges, strawberries and bananas.

The incidence of gastrointestinal complications is low after cardiopulmonary bypass, occurring in about 1% of patients, but the mortality is high. Gastrointestinal bleeding (40%) is the most frequent complication, followed by pancreatitis at 34%. Other complications include cholecystitis (11%), duodenal ulcer (8%), ischaemic bowel (5%) and diverticulitis (2%). Complications are more likely to occur in patients undergoing procedures with longer pump and cross-clamp times (e.g. valve and coronary artery bypass grafts). Patients requiring re-do procedures and the use of intra-aortic balloon pumping are known to have an increased incidence of gastrointestinal complications (2.5–12 times more). These complications may not be immediately identified, so starting oral fluids and diet should be gradual. Initially sips of water may be offered, followed by larger volumes of clear fluid, unrestricted fluid and light diet. Once fluids are taken without any problem, the intravenous fluid can be discontinued, and this usually occurs within 24 hours of surgery. Restricting oral fluids in the early postoperative period does not decrease the incidence of vomiting and nausea, but delays the first bout of vomiting; however, Martin et al. (1990) reported that restricting oral intake for the first 8 hours significantly decreases the incidence of emesis.

Diet can start as soon as the patient is able to swallow and tolerate fluids. A light diet is initially encouraged, which progresses to a normal diet for the patient as soon as possible. This provides a good opportunity for nursing staff to provide guidance on a healthy diet. Patients usually experience a depressed appetite after surgery, and the emphasis should be on encouraging the patient to eat. Ultimately a fat-reduced diet should be striven for, but the patient should be assisted in making an informed decision rather than be given a restricted choice.

Loss of appetite is a common complaint in the immediate postoperative period. To reduce the risks of anorexia or malnutrition, patients should be encouraged to eat any food. Once normal appetite returns (which could take up to 4 weeks), the patient should be directed and advised on the advantages of a low-fat or healthy diet. In giving advice on diet, the nurse must be conscious of cholesterol levels. Lipid-lowering tablets should be recommenced as soon as possible after surgery. Patients whose cholesterol levels were observed to be raised preoperatively, but who were not previously on lipid-lowering therapy, should have fasting cholesterol levels taken at a later date before the decision to start lipid-lowering medication is made.

Postoperative nausea and vomiting

A more frequent complication after anaesthesia for any surgery is postoperative nausea and vomiting. This may be the result of hunger, or a reaction to the anaesthetic agents or opioid-derived analgesia. Some common factors in relation to postoperative nausea and vomiting have been observed and are summarised in Table 7.1. The incidence of nausea and vomiting is greatest among children aged up to 16 years and reduces into adulthood. Women appear to have an increased incidence, but no reason has been established, although many believe that it is linked to the female hormones (Beatie et al., 1993). There is a positive relationship between body weight and nausea. Again, no one theory has been confirmed, but the link has been suggested that soluble anaesthetic may accumulate in the adipose tissue. This anaesthetic is released slowly, prolonging the after effects (Kenny, 1994).

Increased anxiety appears to result in a higher incidence of nausea, but the reasons are unknown. Patients who present with a history of

Table 7.1 Factors affecting the incidence of postoperative nausea and vomiting in cardiac patients

Age
Sex
Obesity
Anxiety
Past medical history
Postoperative fasting
Premedication
Anaesthetic agents
Length of operation
Postoperative pain
Dizziness

motion sickness have a threefold increase in reports of nausea, and patients with medical conditions relating to delayed gastric emptying are also likely to experience nausea. Food itself is not an emetic stimulus, but some studies with animals have demonstrated that food induces abdominal vagal afferent activity and this, combined with anaesthesia, is sufficient to produce emesis. An incidence has yet to be linked to preoperative fasting (Tate and Cook, 1996).

Premedication is considered to be one of the main factors in contributing to the variation in incidence of postoperative nausea and vomiting, with morphine being identified as a significant risk factor. The longer the operation, the greater the incidence of nausea, but this relationship has not been clearly identified and is thought to result from an increased administration of potentially emetic drugs.

Although nausea and vomiting may be viewed as mere inconvenience by the health-care professional, to the patient – particularly during the period of intubation – it can be painful and distressing.

Antiemetics are administered as a prophylactic measure when nausea or vomiting may be anticipated, and as symptom control when a patient complains of nausea or when a patient is already vomiting. It is most often given in response to the complaint of nausea or as a result of vomiting and on these occasions the oral route of administration is not generally recommended. The following are antiemetics commonly used in cardiac surgery.

Butyrophenones (e.g. haloperidol, droperidol)

These act on the chemoceptive trigger zones and are useful for emesis induced by drugs. They are commonly given as part of a premedication.

Phenothiazines (e.g. prochlorperazine)

These drugs act by blocking several types of receptors – dopamine, muscarinic, H_1 and α-adrenergic. They are most useful in metabolic disturbances, terminal illness, opioid administration, radiotherapy and chemotherapy.

Dopamine antagonists (e.g. metoclopramide)

The actions of these drugs result in increased tone of the stomach muscle and increased gastric emptying. They are effective in the treatment of postoperative vomiting, radiotherapy and drug-induced vomiting.

Drug treatment should be timed so that antiemetics are given 20–30 min before a vomiting stimulus is encountered. Drugs should be administered regularly to maintain therapeutic blood levels until the stimulus is no longer active. Patients experiencing postoperative nausea in the early stages of their recovery may be afraid to resume eating and, although they do not appear malnourished or emaciated, loss of appetite over a prolonged period may result in malnutrition and depression. It is common practice to administer antiemetics following periods of vomiting or in patients complaining of nausea. However, evidence suggests that the effectiveness of antiemetics is enhanced if routinely given prophylactically for the first 48 hours after surgery. The symptoms of nausea may continue for up to 4 weeks after surgery (Johnson, 2000).

Control of gastrointestinal bleeding

One of the complications of surgery that is enhanced by mechanical ventilation is the development of gastric ulcer, which if left unchecked could rupture with subsequent life-threatening bleeding. The use of acid-reducing medication during a ventilated period is thought to reduce the risk of ulcer formation. Intravenous ranitidine is frequently prescribed for the duration of mechanical ventilation. If the patient has a history of gastric ulceration, the patient's usual medication is resumed as soon as oral fluids are resumed. Some surgeons prefer to continue with prophylactic medication such as ranitidine for several weeks after discharge.

Intravenous fluids

Intravenous hydration is initially achieved by the infusion of 5% dextrose via the triple-lumen central venous pressure (CVP) line. The priority in the care of these lines is maintaining adequate hydration and fluid balance, and avoiding the complications of central cannulation, of which infection is one of the most frequent. A peripheral cannula is also sited for the administration of colloids. The first plastic peripheral intravenous device was developed in 1945. Then it was usually considered necessary to contact a surgeon to insert the device. In 1950, a simplified intravenous device was introduced consisting of a plastic catheter over a steel needle. Today the insertion of peripheral cannulae is likely to be carried out by medical or nursing staff. Most peripheral cannulae should be removed or replaced after 72 hours, when the incidence of thrombophlebitis increases dramatically (Campbell, 1998).

Complications relating to central lines can occur during insertion, while indwelling or on removal. Table 7.2 highlights the complications most frequently encountered. Pneumothorax is one of the most serious and potentially life-threatening complications of a central line and occurs mainly with the subclavian approach, the rate of incidence ranging from 0% to 6% (Arora and Trikha, 1999). To minimise the incidence, on return from the operating room patients should have a chest radiograph to confirm positioning. Ideally, fluids should not be infused until the position has been confirmed, but this is not always an available option, particularly if the patient is unstable and requires chemical cardiac support.

Venous air embolism can occur at any time from insertion to a few days after removal. The incidence is unknown but is thought to carry a mortality rate of between 29% and 50% (Nielan and Nyguist, 1991). Action should be directed at prevention by way of placing the patient in the Trendelenburg position on insertion (increases central pressure above atmospheric pressure), maintaining a closed system during treatment and positioning the patient flat in the Trendelenburg position on removal.

The incidence of arterial puncture varies from 0.9% to 2.8% (Arora and Trikha, 1999). Haematoma formation is mainly caused by accidental

Table 7.2 Complications related to central venous catheters

Insertion	Pneumothorax
	Venous air embolism
	Arterial puncture
	Haematoma formation
	Catheter misplacement
	Cardiac tamponade
	Cardiac arrhythmias
	Thoracic duct injury
Post-insertion	Superficial thrombophlebitis
	Thrombosis
	Systemic bacteraemia and fungaemia
	Infection
	Thrombus and fibrin sheath formation
	Lipid accumulation
	Precipitation of medication
	Pinch-off syndrome
	Catheter fracture
Post-removal	Air embolism
	Haemorrhage

arterial puncture. Most haematomas are insignificant, but a minority may compromise a patient's airway or paralyse the vocal cords as a result of nerve compression. The incidence of perforation-related cardiac tamponade when a central venous catheter is *in situ* is reported as 0.2% (Jiha et al., 1996), but misdiagnosis may make this figure inaccurate. Cardiac tamponade in relation to central lines is where the vein, right atrium or right ventricle wall is perforated as a result of erosion by the central catheter. This perforation allows excess fluid to be present in the pericardial sac. The risk can be minimised, if not eliminated, by ensuring that the catheter tip is placed outside the cardiac silhouette on the chest radiograph. If the tip of the catheter touches the cardiac wall, cardiac arrhythmias are likely to occur. Thoracic duct injury is a rare complication seen when a left-sided subclavian approach is used.

Insertion of central lines allows direct access for micro-organisms that can enter the insertion site and bloodstream. Infection is the most common complication with central lines, and catheter-related infection is recognised as a significant clinical problem, the incidence of infection ranging from 4% to 8% (Drewitt, 2000). This figure may be higher in the presence of total parental nutrition infusion (Arora and Trikha, 1999). The organisms commonly associated with infection are coagulase-negative staphylococci, *Staphylococcus aureus* and *Candida* species. Most infections are caused by skin micro-organisms that invade the transcutaneous wound; these can be substantially reduced if care is given to aseptic technique during insertion and after-care. It is also known that the risk of infection increases with the duration of placement.

The site of insertion may influence the likelihood of subsequent infection. The most commonly accessed site is the internal jugular vein, but this carries a higher risk of infection than subclavian veins, which demonstrate a higher risk of surgical complications. Other sites are supraclavicular, antecubital fossa veins and femoral veins, although the last are associated with a high rate of infection and should be avoided where possible.

It has been proposed that prophylactic antibiotics given at the time of insertion may reduce the infection rates, and indeed prophylactic cover is usually maintained until such lines are removed. Some centres advocate the use of topical antiseptic or antibiotic/antimicrobial ointments, but these agents have the disadvantage of encouraging the development of resistant staphylococci.

There is conflicting evidence about catheter care, with regard to both method and frequency of dressings. Gauze dressings do not protect the insertion site from moisture or allow it to be easily inspected, and require at least daily dressing change. Transparent dressings, although allowing for easy observation, can increase the number of bacteria around the insertion site. However, this likelihood is connected to the permeability of different dressings to moisture vapour. Insertion sites covered by transparent dressings should be changed as clinically indicated, i.e. when the dressing is no longer intact or when moisture has collected underneath it.

For the small percentage of patients requiring a prolonged period of CVP monitoring, replacement of the catheter must also cause debate, and the frequency of replacement may depend on the manufacturer's instructions. Some institutions re-site central catheters at regular intervals, but most replace catheters based on the condition of the patient, the function of the catheter at the time, and the virulence of the infecting organisms.

Central venous complications, such as occlusion and thrombosis, have the potential to be detrimental to the well-being of the patient. Occlusion can occur from fibrin sheath formation, precipitates of medication, thrombosis, catheter malposition or external compression. Thrombosis occurs from mechanical, chemical or bacterial causes, such as inadequate flow through the catheter or infusion of irritant solutions. Intermittent use may also result in thrombosis formation, so regular flushing is advocated. This can be achieved by way of a continuous heparinised flush, which is necessary if CVP monitoring is required, or intermittent flushing when infusions are discontinued, after bolus injections, or every 12 hours if not otherwise used.

Removal of central lines is not without hazards. A devastating complication is an air embolism, which could result in permanent neurological deficits or slowly resolving deficits. This can be avoided by placing the patient in the Trendelenburg position, lying supine or slightly head down. If the patient is breathless and unable to tolerate these positions, the recumbent position can be used. The patient should perform the Valsalva manoeuvre (forced expiration with the mouth closed) or expiration if the patient is unable to perform this technique. Haemorrhage can occur if there is insufficient occlusion at the vacated insertion site. An occlusive dressing should be placed over the insertion site and left in place for 24 hours. When clinical signs of infection are present, the tip of the catheter should be sent for culture and sensitivity.

Extended periods of ventilation and critical illness cause muscular dystrophy, which includes respiratory musculature. This is augmented by stress-related gluconeogenesis, in which muscle stores of protein are depleted and the protein is used as an alternative energy source. The resulting impaired respiratory muscle function will interfere with effective weaning from ventilation and may even increase the period of ventilation. Therefore, if there is a delay in the weaning of the patient from mechanical ventilation, nutrition, either enteral or parental, should be started as soon as possible. In 1993, McCain predicted that the overall incidence of malnutrition in an intensive care setting could be as high as 50%. Poor nutritional status will be reflected in delayed wound healing and reduced immune status.

Enteral nutrition (where possible) is the therapy of choice because it maintains mucosal integrity, increases blood flow to the gut, minimises septic complications by promoting bacterial translocation, promotes normal gut function and may increase survival. It is also relatively cheap compared with other means of nutrition. Nasogastric feeding is therefore the choice of artificial nutritional support in patients who have a functioning gastrointestinal tract. There is sustained evidence that the gastrointestinal barrier function is compromised by the absence of nutrients in the gut, and enteral nutrition reduces colonisation of the upper gastrointestinal tract, consequently reducing the incidence of nosocomial pneumonia. Once the patient is regarded as being at risk nutritionally, nutritional requirements should be assessed by a dietitian on an individual basis, taking into account the following: clinical condition, disease state, the intended aim of nutritional support and whether an enteral feed is to act as the sole source of nutrition.

Feeding is usually commenced by a Ryle's tube, once its correct positioning has been checked. There are several methods of checking the placement of the tube, including air auscultation, visual observation of the aspirate, testing the pH of the aspirate and abdominal radiograph.

Air auscultation

A total of 20–30 ml air is rapidly injected through the tube while auscultating over the stomach. The sound of air gushing in the stomach should indicate correct tube placement, but this alone may not be a wholly accurate test.

Visual inspection of aspirate

This is not an accurate method because the fluid could be wrongly identified as gastric aspirate when it may be straw-coloured or yellow pleural fluid from malpositioned tubes.

Testing the pH of the aspirate

If fluid can be aspirated from the tube, its pH can be checked using blue litmus or pH test paper (blue paper turns bright red). However, in some instances, the pH of the gastric fluid may be elevated, e.g. if patients are receiving antacids, or H_2-receptor antagonists. Generally, however, this is a good indicator if not totally foolproof.

Abdominal radiograph

This is the only accurate and totally reliable test for checking nasogastric tube placement, but it may result in exposing the patient to X-rays. The tube placement can usually be determined by using pH testing and air auscultation. A radiograph is indicated if there is any doubt. The tip of the nasogastric tube should be within the stomach beyond the cardiac sphincter.

The feeding regimen should include a fasting period, because this has been shown to reduce the incidence of nosocomial pneumonia, although this has also been questioned. During nasogastric feeding, it is prudent to nurse the patient in a semi-head-raised position (34–40°) because this helps to discourage reflux and aspiration. Patients are at risk of aspiration during procedures such as aggressive physiotherapy and postural drainage. If initial feeding is well tolerated, and is likely to continue over a prolonged period, the Ryle's tube can be replaced by a fine-bore nasogastric tube to promote patient comfort and reduce nasal/pharyngeal complications. When feeding has commenced, the tube placement should be checked daily before a feed is restarted. The tube should be taped comfortably, but securely, on to the nose and sheet for comfort, and it is advisable to change the tape daily. Cleaning the nose with mild soap and water removes grease and thoroughly drying the nose encourages adherence of the tape. The nostrils should be kept clean, dry and free from crusts or discharge.

The nasogastric tube should be flushed with 20–30 ml water at the following times: before starting, interrupting or stopping a feed, if tube blockage is suspected; after aspirating gastric contents because aspirate will cause the feed to curdle in the tube, and before and after administering medicines. Generally, it is thought that early enteral nutrition is as good as total parental nutrition (TPN) in maintaining or improving nutritional status. Enteral nutrition reduces the incidence of septic complications compared with TPN.

Problems have been identified with the use of wide-bore (Ryle's) tubes. They are prone to hardening as a result of the effect of the gastric acid, and may render the oesophageal sphincter incompetent, causing the complications of gastric reflux, oesophageal erosion and stricture formation. It is often advocated therefore to replace the large-bore tubes with smaller Clinifeed-type, fine-bore, nasogastric tubes as soon as possible. This procedure may avoid the complications and also prevent the need to replace the tube every 7 days.

However, fine-bore tubes are not free of complications, and are seen to correlate with bronchial, peritoneal and intracranial placement (Colagiovanni, 1999), and many of the incidents are invariably caused by the stylette used in insertion. With the increased use of fine-bore feeding tubes, malpositioning in the airway, even in the presence of a cuffed ET tube is possible, with the potentially serious consequences of pneumonia, hydropneumothorax and lung abscess if unrecognised. The presence of an ET tube is thought to contribute to feeding tube misplacement. In addition, the tests previously described to determine correct placement may be misleading or unreliable with narrow-bore tubes. Aspiration is unreliable and frequently impossible because these tubes have a tendency to collapse when a negative pressure is applied to them. The tube itself can become easily displaced and position can be confirmed only with a radiograph. A radiograph is advocated after any period of vomiting and retching. If tube position requires confirming before commencing a feed, the patient may be exposed to additional X-rays. Crushed medication should not be delivered via a fine-bore tube and a suspension alternative should be sought.

Critically ill patients are often thought to have a paralytic ileus resulting from a decrease in gastric absorption, which is caused by a reduction in smooth muscle contraction, although they may still be able to tolerate nutrition by the nasogastric route regardless of the presence of bowel sounds. Occasionally, patients may not be able to absorb enteral feeds and this may lead to abdominal distension, regurgitation, vomiting and possible pulmonary aspiration. Causes for the delay in gastric emptying include the administration of opioids, the use of low-dose dopamine and possible catecholamine infusions, poor gastric perfusion, electrolyte and fluid abnormality, and the response to stress and pain.

The most frequently cited amount of residual volume that should cause concern is 150–200 ml in gastric feeding. When this occurs, it is possible to reduce the feed rate to 10 ml/h, the minimum rate necessary for gastrointestinal mucosal protection, and medical advice should be sought on whether total parental nutrition should be commenced. Gastrokinetic agents, e.g. metoclopramide, can be given in an attempt to speed the return of gastric emptying.

Nausea, abdominal distension, and discomfort and diarrhoea are often associated with the administration of enteral feeds. These occurrences, particularly diarrhoea, can be minimised by administering the feed at room temperature, because cold feed could act as an irritant to the intestinal mucosa and increase gut mobility; it is often common practice to discontinue the enteral feed. Diarrhoea can be controlled by the addition of roughage to the feeds, and ensuring that the patient is not constipated and displaying overflow. Diarrhoea frequently occurs in critically ill patients, but it should not be assumed to be caused by feed intolerance because there are many other causes, including antibiotic therapy and hypoalbuminaemia. Therefore, until the aetiology has been clearly established, feeding should not be disrupted.

In patients in whom parental nutrition is indicated (i.e. in the presence of oesophageal obstruction or impaired gastric emptying, or patients with high risk of aspiration), it should be via a peripherally inserted central catheter, or by a dedicated lumen of a freshly inserted central line (within 24 hours and previously unused). If high-dose propofol is in use, this should be considered when calculating fat intake. Parental nutrition requires increased nursing intervention with regard to metabolic, mechanical and infectious complications, and may necessitate the instigation of insulin therapy. Plasma protein levels, particularly serum albumin, are sometimes used inappropriately as a guide to nutritional status. However, albumin levels fall as part of an acute phase response to illness and are not a reliable measure (Reilly, 1998).

Biochemical and haematological investigations should be made. Urea, electrolyte and phosphate levels should initially be monitored to assess hydration state and detect electrolyte/phosphate imbalance until a stable regimen has been devised. Raised serum levels of urea and sodium could be indicative of dehydration and more fluid may be required. Hyperglycaemia could occur, but is an uncommon complication of nasogastric feeding. However, patients with mild or undiagnosed diabetes or impaired renal function are at risk (Bockus, 1991). Patients with diabetes should be monitored according to their normal routine when a change in diet is experienced.

Tube feeding can be discontinued when the patient is taking approximately half his or her requirements orally.

Management of the patient with diabetes

Re-starting insulin should be delayed until central normothermia has been restored or rebound hypoglycaemia may occur. In a patient who is ventilated and sedated, the physical signs associated with hypoglycaemia may become masked.

The stress response to surgery involves an immediate release of hormones that cause a rise in blood glucose levels. In a patient with type 1 diabetes (i.e. with absolute insulin deficiency), these effects can lead to hyperglycaemia, ketoacidosis, electrolyte disturbances and protein catabolism. In a patient with type 2 diabetes (i.e. with compromised insulin secretions and insulin resistance), the effects are less marked but, without adequate treatment, severe hyperglycaemia and increased protein losses can still occur. With persistent hyperglycaemia, wound healing can become impaired and the risk of local infection may increase.

There is no agreement on the frequency of capillary blood glucose monitoring, although the stability of the previous blood glucose control and difficulty of surgery should dictate frequency. A target whole blood glucose of 5–10 mmol/l is usually recommended. In the initial postoperative period, hourly estimations may be required, particularly during the hypothermic period.

For patients with type 1 or type 2 diabetes normally treated with insulin, reversion to maintenance insulin therapy needs care. The first light breakfast after surgery should be eaten while the intravenous infusion of insulin continues, to check that the meal is tolerated. Patients who normally take a subcutaneous bolus regimen can be given their usual dose before the next meal, but the intravenous insulin infusion should be continued for an hour, or at least until the meal is completed, to allow for absorption of the subcutaneous insulin. For patients normally on twice daily insulin (who do not take a lunch-time dose), the normal subcutaneous dose can be given before the evening meal. If glycaemic control is not maintained after reinstating the normal insulin, specialised advice should be sought, and intravenous insulin may be required further.

Patients with type 2 diabetes, normally treated with oral hypoglycaemic drugs, but given intravenous insulin during surgery, may temporarily need intermittent subcutaneous insulin before returning to their usual regimen (e.g. as a result of a prolonged stress response after major surgery). It is important to establish how stability is usually achieved, how control is monitored and the carer's knowledge and ability.

References

Arora MK, Trikha A (1999) Central venous catheterisation: routes and complications. *J Anaesthesiol Clin Pharmacol* **15**: 117–19.

Beatie WS, Lindbald R, Buckley DN, Forrest JB (1993) Menstruation increases the risk of nausea and vomiting after laparoscopy. *Anesthesiology* **78**: 272–6.

Bockus S (1991) Troubleshooting your tube feeding. *Am J Nursing* **49**(5): 24–8.

Campbell L (1998) IV related phlebitis, complications and length of hospital stay: 1. *Br J Nursing* **7**: 1304–12.

Colagiovanni L (1999) Taking the tube. *Nursing Times* **95**(21): 63–71.

Drewitt SR (2000) Complications of central venous catheters: nursing care. *Br J Nursing* **9**: 466–78.

Jiha JG, Weinberg GL, Laurito CE (1996) Intraoperative cardiac tamponade after central venous cannulation. *Anesth Analg* **82**: 664–5.

Johnson K (2000) Use of telephone follow-up for post cardiac surgery patients. *Intensive Crit Care Nursing* **16**: 144–50.

Kenny GNC (1994) Risk factors for post-operative nausea and vomiting. *Anaesthesia* **49**(suppl): 6–10.

McCain R (1993) A sensible approach to the nutritional support of mechanically ventilated critically ill patients. *Intensive Care Med* **19**: 129–39.

Martin T, Whitney L, Seidl-Friedman J, Nicolson S, Schreiner M (1990) Drinking before discharging children from day surgery: is it necessary? *Anesthesiology* **73**(A): A1122.

Nielan JB, Nyguist J (1991) Subclavian catheter removal. *J Intraven Nurse* **14**: 114–18.

Reilly H (1998) Enteral feeding: an overview of indications and techniques. *Br J Nursing* **7**: 510–21.

Tate S, Cook H (1996) Post operative nausea and vomiting 1: physiology and aetiology. *Br J Nursing* **5**: 962–73.

CHAPTER 8

Wound drainage and urinary care

Chest drainage

Two of the most common and potentially life-threatening complications following cardiac surgery are cardiac tamponade and haemorrhage. Management of chest drains and close monitoring of the patient can both prevent these conditions and allow for early recognition of the complication. The priority in management is to reverse the process, and this is usually achieved by opening the sternal wound (emergency sternotomy) to remove fluid clots and to identify the source of the blood loss. Reoperation occurs in 1–2% of patients undergoing myocardial revascularisation (Pierce et al., 1991).

Cardiac tamponade

Cardiac tamponade is the pathological accumulation of fluid within the pericardial sac that compresses venous return and reduces cardiac output by preventing adequate cardiac filling. The fluid exerts pressure that is transmitted across the myocardium, increasing ventricular end-diastolic pressure and impairing ventricular filling during diastole.

Signs and symptoms

- Decreased tissue perfusion/cold peripheries related to low cardiac output
- Confusion
- Hypotension
- Tachycardia
- Distension of neck veins/raised jugular venous pressure
- Reduced urine output.

This complication usually occurs in the initial hours after surgery, when a sudden change in the cardiovascular status can be seen in addition to a change in chest drainage. However, tamponade can occur over a longer period of days and has a less acute presentation. In these instances, the drains have usually been removed, cardiovascular deterioration is less well defined and the neurological manifestations may be more evident. Sudden cardiac arrest could occur – usually pulseless electrical activity (PEA).

Diagnosis involves a chest radiograph, cardiac echocardiogram and, on occasions, isoprenaline to test the reaction of the heart to increased myocardial demand. Normally the administration of isoprenaline would result in an increased heart rate. In cardiac tamponade, the heart may not respond to this trigger.

Care of mediastinal chest drains

Following cardiac surgery, one or two chest drainage tubes are customarily left in place in the mediastinum. By preventing fluid accumulation in the tube(s), cardiac tamponade can be prevented because it allows the amount of bleeding from the surgical site to be monitored. A pleural drain may also be in position, particularly following coronary artery bypass grafts (CABGs) using the internal mammary artery (IMA). The following are the nurse's responsibilities in caring for a patient with mediastinal chest drains:

- maintaining chest tube patency
- ensuring correct positioning of the chest tubes
- maintaining accurate records of drainage
- ensuring correct removal.

Chest tube patency

This is a major responsibility for a nurse caring for a cardiac surgical patient. Patency can be achieved by the following:

- gravity and suction
- fanfolding/squeezing
- stripping ('milking' for the purposes of this description).

Gravity and suction

This should always be the main method of ensuring chest tube patency. These two elements are usually sufficient to expel air or blood from the cavity. This method can be enhanced, by keeping the tubing coiled on the bed near the patient. This increases the drainage of the chest cavity, because a chest tube with a dependent loop requires more pressure to evacuate air, and gravity is hindered.

If the chest tubes are connected to a sump (cardiotomy reservoir) bottle −5 kPa of suction should be applied. This is not usually required if the chest tubes are connected to an underwater seal bottle, unless specifically requested by medical staff.

Fanfolding/squeezing

If clots are apparent in the chest tubes, and appear to be hindering drainage, these can be evacuated through the application of pressure just above the clot by squeezing or fanfolding the tube. This procedure should not be undertaken if clots are not troublesome, because this action increases negative pressure and can promote bleeding.

Stripping/milking

This involves using a mechanical stripper. Re-expansion of compressed tubing produces a transiently high level of negative pressure. This pulse of suction drains the air or liquid in the tubing into the drainage unit. This high negative pressure will remain in the tubing until it is replaced by an equivalent volume of air or liquid.

Concern has been raised about possible injury to the intrathoracic tissue adjacent to the chest tubing eyelets from this negative pressure. There is evidence to show that it encourages both tissue entrapment in the eyelets and bleeding. This technique should, therefore, be employed only in the event of a suspected cardiac tamponade, when slight movement of a clot may improve a patient's condition until more aggressive treatment can be commenced. The nurse should therefore observe the viscosity of the drainage, in addition to the amount, before determining the method to be used in ensuring patency.

Correct positioning and safety

On arrival back to the intensive care/recovery area, a chest radiograph should be ordered as soon as the patient's condition stabilises, unless otherwise indicated by medical staff. Drains are marked with radio-opaque strips interrupted at the position of the side holes. The frequency of radiographs taken to monitor the position and effectiveness of drains is a matter of debate. Some centres advocate daily radiographs, but the presence of a drain for drainage purposes makes a radiograph redundant, and they should be ordered only after a clinical change in the patient. The drainage bottle should be connected to low-pressure suction (−3 kPa to −5 kPa) unless otherwise stated.

If more than one chest drain is present, they should be labelled to indicate their position. This may prevent removal of the wrong drain. If drainage ceases, the tubing should be inspected for kinking as well as for clotting. The drainage bottles should always be kept lower than the patient's chest.

On return from the operating room, and after position changes, the connections in the tubing should be checked to ensure that they are secure. Dressings should be checked daily for signs of infection or bleeding, and changed accordingly. Two drainage clamps should be kept at the bedside for use should disconnection occur. If disconnection does occur, medical staff should be informed and the patient's respiratory status observed. Immediate reconnection is required. If the drains are in place for a prolonged period, and the patient is conscious, arm and shoulder exercises should be advocated to prevent stiffness and discomfort. The patient should have good pain control at all times. Cardiotomy drains are usually removed by two people on the first postoperative day when drainage is minimal. Most purse-string sutures – ties sealing the drain tract – can be removed after 48 hours.

Chest drainage should be observed continuously and recorded on an hourly basis for the first 4 hours after return from the operating room, when it is not unusual to observe 400 ml of drainage. This should subside and the frequency of documentation can be reduced when drainage becomes minimal, i.e. < 20 ml/h. The number of drains and how patency is maintained should be documented in the nursing care plan. It is also good practice to note the viscosity of the drainage. If drainage appears to be excessive, several measures can be instigated in an attempt to minimise it.

The patient's haemodynamic status should be stabilised. This may mean the introduction of vasodilators to maintain normotension and prevent shivering. Uncontrolled hypertension may put pressure on any internal sutures. Until haemodynamic stability is achieved, the patient should remain sedated. Positive end-expiratory pressure (PEEP) can be introduced into the ventilatory system. This has the beneficial effect of compressing mediastinal blood vessels. However, this therapy should be implemented with caution: the introduction of more positive pressure may have an adverse effect on haemodynamic stability.

Haemoglobin, haematocrit, platelet and monitoring of partial thromboplastin time (PTT) is carried out postoperatively. Bleeding from chest drains may indicate that the patient needs a blood transfusion, although blood is prescribed based on the Hb and haematocrit count, as well as on the patient's clinical status. Patient Hb should be maintained above 10. Although this appears low, the patient is likely to experience some degree of haemodilution after cardiopulmonary bypass and, when fluid balance has returned to normal, the Hb returns to normal levels. Alternative measures such as plasma expanders and artificial blood may sometimes be necessary.

If a patient shows signs of haemorrhage on return, it could be because the heparin used in bypass has not been reversed satisfactorily, and in these instances a bolus of protamine sulphate could be administered. In addition, in patients receiving blood drained from the bypass machine, the blood is likely to be contaminated with heparin, so a covering dose of protamine is advantageous. Some patients have been known to have a reaction to protamine, and this usually develops as hypotension within 10 min of administration. To reduce the chances of a reaction, it is recommended that protamine is administered by a slow intravenous infusion during a 5- to 15-min period and the American Hospital Formulary Service recommends that no more than 50 mg of the drug is administered in any 10-min period.

Platelet infusion should be considered for the bleeding patient if the platelet count is less than 100×10^9/L, and depending on the degree of the bleeding. Platelet function is impaired by the bypass process, and platelet numbers are reduced as a consequence of haemodilution by the pump prime. Platelets should be given if levels are between 20 and 30×10^9/L even if bleeding is not in evidence because spontaneous bleeding may develop. Fresh frozen plasma (FFP) contains all the clotting factors apart from platelets, and this is the best option in the presence of a normal haematocrit. If the haematocrit is less than 28%, whole blood should be considered.

Colloids are used as a plasma substitute for short-term replacement of fluid volume, while the cause of the problem is being addressed (e.g. stopping bleeding). These solutions can be blood products (human albumin solution, plasma protein fraction) or synthetic (Haemaccel, Gelofusine). Albumin is used in hypovolaemia and hypoalbuminaemia because it is believed to be effective in replacing volume and supporting colloid oncotic pressure. However, albumin is also believed to have anticoagulation properties, inhibiting platelet aggregation and enhancing the inhibition of factor Xa and antithrombin III. This anticoagulation activity may be detrimental to patients experiencing haemorrhage hypovolaemia.

Blood transfusion

The logical indication for prescribing blood is to increase oxygen delivery by the blood to the tissues. Patients with a substantial blood loss can benefit from blood transfusion. However, most perioperative transfusions are given to raise the Hb above levels which, although below normal, are not immediately life threatening. Some stored blood contains sodium citrate which uses the body's ionised calcium ions and causes citrate toxicity. The may present as muscle tremor, tetanus, circulatory depression and ECG changes caused by hypocalcaemia. Calcium gluconate may be given intravenously after alternate units of blood to compensate for this.

Blood for transfusion should not be removed from a temperature-controlled storage area, until a maximum of 30 min before the start of infusion. Blood not used within this time should really be discarded because of the risk of bacterial proliferation. A report produced by the Serious Hazards of Transfusion Steering Group in 1999 (SHOT, 1999) indicated that human errors represent the single greatest risk to patients receiving blood transfusions. Other agents have a place in the treatment of patients with abnormal clotting mechanisms and may minimise the use of allogeneic blood. These are listed in Table 8.1.

If a patient is haemorrhaging and no blood is immediately available, or if the patient has refused a blood transfusion for religious/moral reasons, autotransfused blood can be given. Here, blood that is shed can be re-infused once filtered. Although this may prevent the need for a blood transfusion in the short term, over a long period it can contribute to renal failure; it should therefore be only a short-term solution, and other solutions should be sought, e.g. returning the patient to the operating room.

Urinary function

All patients will have a urinary catheter *in situ* on return from the operating room and this is usually via the urethra. For patients with prostatic problems, which make urethral catheterisation difficult, a suprapubic catheter can be inserted. Hourly measurements are taken until the catheter is removed, in order not only to assess kidney function but also to ensure that an accurate fluid balance is maintained.

Table 8.1 Agents that can be used to minimise the use of allogeneic blood

Agent*	Characteristics
Cryoprecipitate	A rich source of factors I, VII and XII
Ethamsylate (Dicynene)	Reduces capillary bleeding in the presence of normal numbers of platelets. It is believed to correct platelet adhesion
Tranexamic acid (Cyklokapron)	Impairs fibrin dissolution. It inhibits plasminogen activation and fibrinolysis
Aprotinin (Trasylol)	Supplement plasmin inhibitors. It is thought to minimise the derangement of the coagulation system that occurs during cardiopulmonary bypass, and is specifically indicated for this purpose. It is not indicated for reduction of blood loss during cardiac surgery
Desmopressin	This is used when haemorrhage is caused by an acquired defect in the formation of the platelet plug, and deficiency in factor VIII. This facilitates the release of factor VII from tissue sores, thereby improving platelet adherence, lowers the bleeding time and improves haemostasis

*The generic names are given with the proprietary names in parentheses.

Urine output is usually maintained at 0.5–1.0 ml/kg per h. Fluid balance figures need to be collated hourly and infusion rates altered also on an hourly basis to help prevent a gross deficit or an accumulation of fluid. If periods of oliguria occur, it may be prudent to look for kinks in the catheter tubing, assess the patient's bladder, try a bladder lavage or change the catheter. Positioning the catheter to allow free drainage without gravitational loops is also a priority. Attention should be paid to prevent the bag being positioned more than 30 cm below the level of the catheter because this may create negative pressure within the bladder and cause trauma.

Renal failure after cardiopulmonary bypass was very problematic in the initial development of surgery, but it is now thought to occur in around 2% of cases. Preoperative serum creatinine, advanced age and more complicated procedures increase the risk of postoperative renal failure. Low-dose dopamine by continuous intravenous infusion is thought to improve renal function after bypass, and it is usually continued for 24 hours, or until the serum urea and creatinine are within normal limits. Dopamine at 0.5–3 µg/kg per min achieves a specific dopaminergic renal vasodilating action without the inotropic effects achieved at higher doses. Dopamine also causes natriuresis by inhibition of the sodium/

potassium pump within the kidney (Evans, 1998). Inhibition of the sodium/potassium pump may reverse some of the sodium and water retention that occurs in acute renal failure, and decrease the incidence of fluid overload. If the metabolic demands on the nephron can be reduced by the inhibition of the highly active sodium/potassium pumps, the reduced oxygen supply may be better tolerated. Although renal blood flow and urine output are increased in the healthy kidney, there is no clear evidence that 'renal dose' dopamine is able to prevent or reverse developing acute renal failure (Beale and Dihari, 1992; Denton et al., 1996) and dopamine continues to be used at the discretion of the prescribing physician. The dopamine is discontinued and, providing that urinary function has been adequate and urea and electrolytes are within normal limits for the patient, the urinary catheter is also removed.

In some cases, furosemide (frusemide) can be used to stimulate the kidneys and promote urine output, but will be effective only if renal perfusion is adequate. Osmotic diuretic mannitol is sometimes employed to try to restore the urine output but, again, adequate renal perfusion is necessary for any effect.

After surgery a patient should be weighed on a daily basis, with the aim of returning the patient to his or her preoperative weight. Frequently, the patients are oedematous during the initial postoperative days, returning from the operating room 5–10 kg above their preoperative weight (Bojar, 1994), and a good diuresis is usually expected on the patient's initial return from the operating room. During this large diuretic stage, it is important that the central venous pressure (CVP) is monitored to prevent hypovolaemia occurring. The urine may also appear blood stained in the initial period, a symptom called oxyhaemoglobinuria; this results from damage to red blood cells by the cardiopulmonary bypass machine. It usually resolves over a few hours, but a worsening of the symptoms to clearly blood-stained urine requires treatment, usually in the form of 100 ml 10% mannitol.

Renal failure

A complication that can arise as a result of cardiac surgery is acute renal failure. Under normal haemodynamic conditions, the kidneys receive 20–25% of cardiac output but, if this drops, or there is a drop in mean arterial pressure, the glomerular filtration rate drops. A significant reduction in renal blood flow will cause ischaemia to renal tissue over a relatively short period of time, with 25 min or less of ischaemia causing mild reversible injury to renal cells. Ischaemia of 40–60 min results in more severe damage, with recovery taking 2–3 weeks. If ischaemia continues over 60–90 min it usually causes irreversible damage, and at this stage prerenal failure may develop into acute tubular necrosis.

Hypoperfusion leads to a compensatory vasoconstriction in the kidneys, which maintains filtration pressure and urine output. If the circulating volume is restored rapidly, renal function is preserved. However, if hypofusion is prolonged, vasoconstriction can lead to ischaemia within the nephron. Sodium and water retention will also occur in an attempt to maintain perfusion. Eventually the glomerular filtration rate decreases and filtration may cease.

The recognition of renal impairment is not difficult. There is a rise in serum urea and creatinine, and there may be an associated rise in serum potassium. A metabolic acidosis usually occurs. Urine output usually diminishes and may often cease. Occasionally, the patient continues to pass urine, but the quality is poor and waste clearance is inadequate to prevent a deteriorating biochemistry. It usually occurs over several days, and is related to a specific cause, categorised as prerenal, renal or post-renal (although cardiac patients fall into the first two categories). Whatever the cause, it is treatable, with a variety of interventions, and is reversible unless the patient has an underlying renal problem when the renal physician should be consulted before surgery. Despite this, renal failure continues to carry a high mortality rate (around 50%) and this is often influenced by elderly patients undergoing more complicated surgery.

Classification

Prerenal failure results from a decreased renal blood flow and consequent reduced glomerular filtration rate, which is reversible and not associated with structural damage to the kidney. The patient is oliguric with concentrated urine and elevated plasma urea levels, but responds to correction of the cause with a rapid reversal of oliguria and uraemia. Some have tried to define it by the volume of urine produced. Less than 400 ml of urine in 24 h is used by some authors, but this does not take account of individual characteristics, namely size and weight. A more accurate estimate can be achieved by using body weight (0.5 ml urine/kg per h). It is often referred to as dysfunction rather than failure because it results from diminished renal perfusion and established tissue damage has not occurred. Reduced renal perfusion may be caused by reduced cardiac output as a result of haemorrhage, myocardial infarction, pulmonary embolism or even positive pressure ventilation. The main intervention is rehydration.

Renal failure (intrinsic renal failure) is characterised by damage to the renal parenchyma, resulting in a sudden deterioration of renal function. Prerenal failure progresses to this stage if not treated. The most common cause is acute tubular necrosis (ATN) following ischaemic damage or nephrotoxicity. Patients at risk of developing ATN are those with hypotension, sepsis and trauma, although ATN is most common in patients who have both sepsis and hypotension. There is no time limit with regard to the period of hypotension. Some patients tolerate hypotensive periods for hours without the development of ATN, whereas others need only be hypotensive for minutes. There is evidence, however, that renal tissue damage will occur only if renal blood flow is less than 25–50%.

Postrenal failure is very rare after cardiac surgery, and accounts for only 10% of all cases of acute renal failure, although it is easily diagnosed by ultrasonography and is reversible. Causes include calculi, bladder-neck obstruction, stricture and tumours.

Once the patient is in recognised renal failure with its associated oliguria and raised levels of urea and creatinine, nursing care is aimed at preventing the complication of acute renal failure becoming life threatening. The main treatment in the initial phase is treating the cause. After cardiac surgery this will be maintaining hydration and preventing hypotension.

During this period, hyperkalaemia (serum potassium levels > 5 mmol/l) and metabolic acidosis are common. Clinical problems and nursing interventions are linked with the abnormal physiological volumes, and include symptoms of uraemia (nausea, vomiting, lethargy, pericarditis, coagulopathy) hyperkalaemia, fluid overload and increased susceptibility to infection.

The following are the main nursing considerations.

Diet

This is an important consideration. Tissue damage associated with acute renal failure is often associated with catabolism, when the patient's energy requirements exceed the supply of available carbohydrates, resulting in catabolism (breakdown) of the body's fat and protein stores. Normally an individual requires about 2000 kcal of energy/day, but a patient in catabolic acute renal failure requires more. The energy intake is based on the patient's weight, and given as a ratio of 35 kcal/kg body weight. Involvement of a dietitian in the management of the patient is crucial to prevent malnutrition.

Fluid management

The fluid status of the patient in acute renal failure can be difficult to manage. The standard calculation for daily fluid intake is 500 ml plus the equivalent of the previous day's urine output. The 500 ml is representative of the insensible loss – respiratory, faecal and perspiration. It is important to note that losses can be increased if the patient is pyrexial, has diarrhoea or is vomiting. Most patients will develop renal failure while in the intensive care/high dependency environment. These patients will have their fluid balance calculated hourly, and replacement is often based on the previous hour's urine output with the addition of 30 ml to accommodate the insensible loss. The replacement fluid must take into account any intravenous infusion or oral intake.

The most accurate method of fluid balance assessment is through daily weighing – 1 kg equals 1000 ml – so any increases in weight should correspond to an increase in fluid retention. It may not be possible to weigh patients who are in bed, although some electric/specialised beds do have a weighing capacity. Weight should be recorded at the same time each day, with the patient wearing similar clothing. Inaccuracies can occur with weighing especially if the scales are poorly maintained and calibrated, but weight combined with fluid balance charts allows for fairly accurate fluid balance assessment and trends can be identified. In the patient without renal impairment, diuretics are administered orally until the preoperative weight is reached and then they are discontinued. Patients requiring diuretics preoperatively for left ventricular failure continue on diuretics for several weeks, especially after valve replacement.

Control of infection

Infection presents problems for patients with acute renal failure both as a causative factor and as a complication. Uraemia causes reduction in the immune status of the patient, increasing the chance of serious infections such as septicaemia and pneumonia. This is exaggerated by a reduction in core temperature, also as a result of uraemia.

Complications of acute renal failure

Hyperkalaemia

Hyperkalaemia, defined as a serum potassium greater than 5.2 mmol/l, is one of the most common complications and the most dangerous. A serum potassium level of more than 6 mmol/l greatly increases the chance of cardiac arrest, and at lower levels may still precipitate dysrhythmias. It can be controlled in a number of ways.

Calcium Resonium may be given orally or rectally. However, if this therapy is used the patient has an increased risk of constipation. When it is administered rectally, the Calcium Resonium should be mixed with methylcellulose, to reduce the risk of faecal impaction.

An infusion of insulin and 50 ml of 50% dextrose will rapidly reduce potassium levels by shifting potassium into the intracellular compartment. This provides only a short-term effect and, once the infusion has been administered, the potassium will shift back into the vascular compartment, raising the serum concentration. The most effective way of controlling potassium is by renal replacement therapy.

Infection

This is a common complication, caused in part by the immunosuppression secondary to uraemia. Infections likely to be encountered are listed in Table 8.2.

Table 8.2 Infection occurring in renal failure

Infection	Causes
Septicaemia	Cannulation
	Venous/arterial catheterisation
Pneumonia	Pulmonary oedema
	Hypostasis
Urinary tract infection	Bedrest
	Urethral catheter (remove if patient is anuric)
	Low urine output

Hypervolaemia

Fluid retention results from electrolyte and water imbalance. The oliguric patient is unable to excrete excess fluid, resulting in volume overload. It can present innocently as dependent tissue oedema, associated with hyponatraemia resulting from sodium dilution by the excess fluid. This dependent oedema presents additional challenges to the nurses with regard to maintaining skin integrity.

Initially, fluid overload is treated with diuretics, especially frusemide, because of its renal vasodilatory effects, supported by dopamine in an attempt to revert oliguric into non-oliguric acute renal failure. When this is achieved, patient management is easier and less expensive in terms of the dialysis required. If the oliguric state persists, fluid removal may be achieved only by renal replacement therapy.

Haemorrhage

Coagulopathies associated with decreased platelet function resulting from the uraemic syndrome represent a problem. This may be compounded by the need to use anticoagulants during dialysis, which increases the risk of gastric bleeding. For this reason, clotting must be reviewed regularly during dialysis treatment. This can be achieved by measuring the activated clotting times (ACTs) at the bedside.

Uraemic pericarditis

Chest pain, especially on inspiration, may indicate uraemic pericarditis. This is associated with a plasma urea in excess of 35 mmol/l and self-resolves once the urea level reduces. It is important that the patient is observed for cardiac tamponade, particularly when heparin is being used to facilitate dialysis. Non-steroidal anti-inflammatory drugs may be required if the patient is symptomatic. The primary control of uraemic pericarditis remains dialysis.

Recovery (diuretic) phase

The course of this is difficult to predict or identify. The most common occurrence is an increase in urine output on a daily basis, although not all patients experience diuresis as renal function improves. It is normal for diuresis to be excessive and it is important that fluid replacement matches urine output. Dehydration is a risk, but overhydration will also perpetuate the large diuresis. The diuresis stabilises at between 5 and 8 days. During the large diuresis, sodium and potassium losses are large, and require frequent monitoring.

Renal replacement therapy

Factors affecting the choice of treatment include patient's diagnosis, availability of resources, and cardiovascular stability and cost; three main options (peritoneal dialysis, haemofiltration or haemodialysis) are regularly used depending on the institution. Fluid overload, acidosis, hyperkalaemia and hyperuraemia are all indications for renal replacement therapy; overhydration may be treated conservatively by fluid restriction. However, in the presence of persistent oliguria or anuria, active fluid removal is necessary to alleviate pulmonary oedema as well as to create space for volume therapy. A urea above 35 mmol/l and/or a plasma creatinine of more than 500 ml/l is usually indicative of the need for intervention, although lower levels may require treatment earlier depending on symptoms. Renal physicians should be instrumental in the decision-making process. The aim of therapy is to provide artificial renal support until recovery eventually occurs.

Peritoneal dialysis

This has become less popular as an intervention for acute renal failure in the last decade. It is simple and inexpensive to set up and run. It can be provided by relatively inexperienced staff if protocols are followed. It does not require the use of large doses of anticoagulants, although the risk of peritonitis and access site leaks restricts its effectiveness. It cannot be used if there is any possibility of recent incision into the abdominal cavity, e.g. use of the gastroepiploic artery during bypass grafts.

Peritoneal dialysis is usually well tolerated by acutely ill patients, but patients who are being ventilated may experience increased respiratory pressures, as a result of fluid pressing on the diaphragm. The nurse needs to be aware of the risk when taking arterial blood samples, the results of which may vary depending on the stage of the fluid exchange. It is usually the treatment of choice where no haemodialysis facilities are available.

Adequate clearances are achieved by exchanges with isotonic dialysate of 1500–2000 ml over short periods of 60–90 min. Short peritoneal dialysis cycles can cause hypokalaemia so monitoring of the plasma potassium level is important. When, and if, hypokalaemia occurs, potassium can be added to the peritoneal dialysis bags. Peritonitis remains the single greatest obstacle in the use of peritoneal dialysis in the acute setting.

Haemodialysis

Haemodialysis is the traditional mode of renal replacement and requires the use of a conventional haemodialysis machine. Treatments are intermittent so control of biochemistry and fluid balance is episodic. This method uses diffusion through a semipermeable membrane down a concentration gradient. Removal of fluid is achieved by ultrafiltration, where the driving force is a hydrostatic pressure gradient. This can be achieved independent of solute transfer. It is the most aggressive of the renal replacement therapies, and is performed by experienced renal nurses. It is used ideally in normotensive patients because it is frequently complicated by cardiovascular instability and episodes of hypotension, which hinder attempts to attain negative fluid balance and contribute to further ischaemic renal injury.

Haemodialysis achieves a better clearance of small solutes, and is therefore more efficient. Once an acute episode is resolved and the patient has solely renal failure as a diagnosis, dialysis is the treatment of choice. It has been proved that small uraemic toxins (urea and creatinine) are more efficiently eliminated with diffuse transport, whereas elimination of larger toxins is achieved better by convective transport.

Haemofiltration

Haemofiltration (filtering of the blood) mimics glomerular filtration, water being forced through a semipermeable membrane by hydrostatic pressure, drawing solutes by convection. The development of this therapy over the last decade has allowed patients with acute renal failure to be cared for in a number of clinical areas without the support of renal nurses. Continuous haemofiltration was first described in the 1960s and Table 8.3 illustrates the types available. Continuous arteriovenous haemofiltration (CAVH) was developed in 1976; continuous venovenous haemofiltration (CVVH) was developed subsequently and is still gaining in popularity.

CVVH

A central vein is cannulated with a double-lumen catheter, the blood for the arterial circuit (i.e. from the patient) being drawn by a pump. Fluid removal through haemofiltration is very efficient, often too efficient. Ultrafiltrate from a new filter may exceed 1 l/h. The haemofilter is

Table 8.3 Types of renal filtration replacement therapies

Type	Abbreviation	Description
Slow continuous filtration	SCU (SCUF)	A technique of continuous ultrafiltration commonly performed without simultaneous fluid replacement
Continuous arteriovenous haemofiltration	CAVH/CAVF	A technique of continuous ultrafiltration with simultaneous fluid replacement. An arteriovenous extracorporeal circuit is used and blood flow generated without the assistance of a mechanical pump
Continuous venovenous haemofiltration	CVVH/CVVF	Ultrafiltration occurring in a veno-venous extracorporeal circuit through which blood is propelled by means of an external blood pump
Continuous ultrafiltration plus intermittent haemodialysis	CUPID	Intermittent haemodialysis performed against a background of continuous ultrafiltration
Continuous arteriovenous haemodiafiltration	CAVHD	Continuous ultrafiltration in an arteriovenous extracorporeal circuit to which a continuous dialysis has been added by the infusion of dialysate into the haemofilter
Continuous venovenous haemodiafiltration	CVVHD	Ultrafiltration and dialysis combined as in CAVHD but performed with the use of a pump-assisted venovenous extracorporeal circuit

unable to mimic the selective reabsorption and this must be mimicked by fluid replacement, which may be achieved by a second function on the blood pump machine.

For the conscious patient, the cardiovascular stability minimises dizziness and confusion. Nausea and vomiting are relatively rare (Woodrow, 1993). Filtration offers greater cardiovascular stability than dialysis, with a 50% reduction in hypotensive episodes compared with dialysis.

If immobility is not a problem, haemofiltration is a relatively comfortable procedure. The limits on mobility are a contraindication to its use, so when a patient recovers from the acute episode that contributed to the development of acute renal failure and is convalescing, therapy is switched to haemodialysis and management of the patient may be overseen entirely by renal physicians. Haemofiltration is effective at creating fluid space for nutrition (especially total parenteral nutrition – TPN) and other therapeutic fluids. The filtration rate and its adjustment depend on the requirement of a negative and positive fluid balance.

The main complications are, therefore, immobility, human error in calculating fluid balance, continuous heparin therapy and heat loss. It is important that the patient's temperature is monitored, although a pyrexia can also be masked.

Inadequate anticoagulation creates irreversible fibrin deposits in filters – reducing efficiency. Clotting may show as darkening of blood, reduction in ultrafiltrate or kinking of lines. The suggested amount of heparin varies, but it is universally acknowledged that there is a need for maintenance of anticoagulation.

Regular checks on the clotting status of the system are required if the filter is to remain efficient for any length of time. If heparin is being used, the ACT should be checked regularly and kept at appropriate levels for the patient. An ACT should be taken to identify a baseline level before starting filtration, and then anticoagulant should be given to keep the clotting time 25–50% longer.

Clotting of the lines and filter is also affected by pump speed. Below 75 ml/min, the risk of stasis within the filter increases the chance of clotting. The presence of high plasma lipid levels increases the coagulability of the blood within the filter, and this is particularly associated with the administration of TPN or high dosages of propofol. When extracorporeal circulations are employed, shear forces are inevitable and may be enhanced by the use of blood pumps. These shear forces have deleterious effects on red blood cells, polymorphs and platelets.

Side effects of artificial kidneys

- Dialysis disequilibrium syndrome: this is characterised by nausea, muscle cramps, hypertension and disorientation, and eventually by seizures and coma. It is caused by cerebral oedema.
- Pulmonary effects: the net effects can be either an improvement in or worsening of the arterial oxygen tension (PaO_2) depending on the patient's cardiopulmonary condition and the technique used. Fluid removal can decrease extravascular lung water, and thus improve gas exchange. Dialysis can also induce hypoxia.
- Haemodynamics: changes in circulating volume and preload.
- Changes in electrolyte concentrations (rhythm disturbances).
- Concentration changes of various vasoactive substances, e.g. catecholamines.

Bowel function

Certain drugs, alteration in diet and immobility can cause constipation which, if it leads to abdominal distension, may interfere with normal diaphragmatic function and ventilatory capacity. Opioids given for analgesia, in addition to limited mobility, are crucial factors. Bulk laxatives or stool softeners can be beneficial and are better than the more aggressive intervention of suppositories and enemas.

Diarrhoea may occur and is often associated with enteral feed intolerance, although other factors, such as reduced gut integrity and overgrowth of antibiotic-resistant organisms, e.g. *Clostridium difficile*, should be considered, even after a relatively short course of antibiotics.

References

Beale R, Bihari D (1992) The management of acute renal failure in the intensive care unit. *Curr Anaesth Crit Care* **3**: 146–7.

Bojar M (1994) *Manual of Peri-operative Care in Cardiac and Thoracic Surgery*. Boston, MA: Blackwell Science. Chap. 8, p. 235.

Denton MD, Chertow GM, Brady HR (1996) 'Renal dose' dopamine for the treatment of acute renal failure: scientific rationale, experimental studies and clinical trials *Kidney Int* **49**: 4–14.

Evans D (1998) Inotropic therapy – current controversies and further directions. *Nursing Crit Care* **3**(1): 8–12.

Pierce J, Piazza D, Naftel D (1991) Effects of two chest tube clearance protocols on drainage in patients after myocardial revascularisation surgery. *Heart Lung* **20**: 125–30.

SHOT (1999) Serious Hazards of Transfusion Steering Group. *Annual Report 1997–1998*. Manchester: SHOT.

Woodrow P (1993) Resource package: haemofiltration. *Intensive Crit Care Nursing* **9**: 95–107.

CHAPTER 9

Hygiene and the prevention of infection

Hygiene

The skin is continually shredding its top layer of epithelial cells. In addition, sweat glands eliminate fluids from the body as sweat and help to regulate body temperature. Sebaceous glands are at the roots of hair follicles and keep the skin and hair soft and supple. Some of the secretions from these glands evaporate, but some dry on the skin and, together with the epithelial debris, form a layer of waste products which, if not removed, will soon block the orifices of the glands and form a breeding ground for pathogenic bacteria and parasites. On exposed parts, dust and dirt will also be deposited. Hygiene provision is therefore part of basic nursing care.

Wound infections

When the surgical incision is closed primarily (as most are), the incision is usually covered with a sterile dressing for 24–48 hours. Beyond 48 hours, reports vary as to whether the incision should be covered by a dressing, and whether showering/bathing is detrimental to healing. When a surgical incision is left open at skin level for a few days before closure (delayed primary closure), the surgeon has usually determined that the patient's condition prevents primary closure (e.g. haemorrhage). In such cases, the incision is packed with a sterile dressing and left untouched until the patient returns to the operating room.

Surgical antimicrobial prophylaxis refers to a brief course of an antimicrobial agent initiated just before an operation starts. It is not an attempt to sterilise tissues, but a critically timed adjunct used to reduce the microbial burden of intraoperative contamination to a level that cannot overwhelm the host defender. It does not prevent infections

caused by postoperative contamination. The agent is usually administered intravenously. Cephalosporins are effective against many Gram-
positive and Gram-negative micro-organisms. In particular, cefazolin is
widely used. The full therapeutic dose should be administered no more
than 30 min before the skin is incised.

Most surgical incisions for cardiac surgery are referred to as class
1/clean. This is defined as an uninfected operative wound in which no
inflammation is encountered, and the respiratory, alimentary, genital or
uninfected urinary tract is not entered. In addition, clean wounds are
primary closed and, if necessary, drained with closed drainage. Operative
incisional wounds after blunt (non-penetrating) trauma are included in
this definition.

The care of wounds and dressings used in wound healing by primary
intention is generally straightforward: a simple dressing is used to cover the
wound; it is applied directly to the wound to provide protection from external contamination and to absorb any exudate. Limbs used for a donor vein
are additionally wrapped in a sterile bandage for the purposes of pressure
and support. Dressings should usually be left *in situ* for 48 hours, but they
are usually replaced in the event of re-exploration for bleeding/tampon-
ade, strike through and external contamination (e.g. vomit).

Chest drains are always inserted after surgery, and occasionally wound
drains are placed at the donor site. The main benefit of using a wound
drain is the obliteration of dead space and the prevention of haematoma
formation underneath the wound. This can, however, be offset by several
disadvantages. Drains can act as bacterial conduits through which conta-
minants can gain access to deep layers of the wound. The presence of a
drain can represent an infection risk, but the risks are reduced with the
use of a closed system. There is also debate about techniques for removing wound drains, in particular the release of the vacuum. The consensus
seems to be that, despite the lack of empirical evidence, it is safer in terms
of tissue trauma to release the vacuum before removing the drains.

Several parameters suggest that the normal pattern of healing is
occurring in primary intention wounds – inflammation for 3–5 days,
epithelialisation within 72 hours, cessation of serous serosanguineous
fluid within 3 days, and the presence of a healing ridge by 7–9 days.
Absence of these processes or inflammation that is prolonged or of both is
indicative of delayed wound healing.

On removing the wound dressing, wound cleaning is usually undertaken. Over the decades several solutions have been in vogue for this
purpose. However, general routine cleaning to remove bacteria and stop

or reduce infection is unlikely to be effective and its roots unfortunately lie in ritualistic practice.

There are instances where wound cleaning is still advocated: to remove visible debris after a wound has initially occurred, to aid assessment, and to remove excessive slough and exudate. Removing exudate will prevent odour and clear the wound bed to aid assessment. Cotton-wool or gauze should not be used for wound cleaning. These materials shed fibres into the wound and the presence of such foreign bodies increases the risk of wound infection. Swabbing is usually carried out with non-woven gauze. It should be confined to skin surrounding the wound. Swabbing over the wound bed can damage newly granulating tissue. If wound cleaning is carried out, it is now acceptable to warm any fluid before cleaning. Cooling the wound inhibits cell mitosis and potentially delays healing. Warm fluid is also more comforting to the patient.

Once the skin edges have sealed, bathing or showering is not likely to present any risk for infection; indeed, studies have failed to show any increased risk of infection when sutured wounds are washed with soap and water from the first postoperative day. Showers are thought to be preferable to a bath because there is less possibility of cross-infection from a previous user.

It has been suggested that, in acute hospitals in the UK 9% of patients have a hospital-acquired infection (Department of Health, 1999). Wound infection after cardiac surgery is a widely documented and recognised complication which can necessitate lengthy and costly hospital admissions. Infections can occur in the sternal wound and following bypass surgery, at the incision of the donor site. The recognised incidence of sternal wound infections, a nosocomial infection, is approximately 2.8 times more costly than it is for patients who have an uncomplicated postoperative course (Ulicny et al., 1990). The reported incidence of sternal wound infection varies, but is reported to be between 0.4% and 7% of patients who have undergone cardiac surgery (Sarr et al., 1984), and it could prolong a hospital stay by 21 days (Weintraub et al., 1989).

The incidence of sternal wound infections may appear small, but it can translate into a large number of patients with a potentially life-threatening complication and devastating chronic effects. The mortality rate attributed to sternal wound infections ranges between 7% and 20% (Hussey et al., 1998). Approximately 10–17% of discharged patients who have experienced sternal wound infections will be readmitted as a result of recurrent sternal infection (Loop et al., 1990). Table 9.1 lists the differing types of sternal wound infections.

Table 9.1 Types of sternal wound infection

Classification	Description
Superficial	Involves skin or subcutaneous tissue, is obvious and treatable
Deep	Involves soft tissues or spaces below the subcutaneous tissue. It may defy conventional methods of diagnosis
Mediastinitis	Infection involving a part of the anatomy other than the incision. The patient is severely ill, with high fever, elevated white cell count, tachycardia, and erythematous, oedematous, tender, sternal wound site. Drainage may or may not be present. Treatment involves antibiotics and a series of débridements. In some cases reconstruction with muscle is required
Sternal osteomyelitis	Infection of the bone

Leg wound infections (after saphenous vein harvesting) may result from poor surgical technique with creation of flaps, failure to eliminate dead space or haematoma formation. It is more common among patients with severe peripheral vascular disease, diabetes and obesity. Although sternal wound infections are undoubtedly more serious, phlebectomy wound infections may result in considerable morbidity and prolonged hospital stay, and Sellick et al. (1991) report that 43.8% of patients have impaired healing at the donor site. Infections are not the only complication associated with saphenous vein harvest incisions. Other reported complications are haematoma, numbness, paraesthesia, lymphoedema, persistent exudate, dermatitis, cellulitis, seroma, skin necrosis, wound separation and rarely amputation (Wipke-Tervis et al., 1996).

The most common pathogen causing wound infection is *Staphylococcus* species with Gram-negative bacilli. The next most common – coagulase-negative staphylococci – is a normal inhabitant of the skin, and these opportunistic pathogens are often multi-resistant.

Signs and symptoms of a wound infection

Infections are usually diagnosed within 30 days of the operative procedure. Heat and redness are usually the first indications that wound healing is problematic and these are accompanied by other signs. The presence of pus is a clear sign of infection in an acute surgical wound. However, in the treated wound, hydrocolloid dressings dissolve to form an exudate similar to pus in appearance and distinction may be difficult. The sudden appearance of increased amounts of exudate in a healing wound may be indicative of infection. This is the result of underlying capillaries dilating as part of the inflammatory response, in order to allow white cells to migrate to the source of infection. As a result, capillaries become leaky, and allow greater quantities of plasma to leak out as well.

Pain may already be present at a surgical wound, but a change in the type or intensity of pain may be an indicator that something is occurring in the wound, and infection should be suspected. The pain may be throbbing in nature, caused by swelling and increased tension, which result from the rise in tissue fluid. Other causal factors for the pain are the presence of toxins and hydrogen ions. There may be a change in the appearance of the granulation tissue. In addition to the increased wetness, infected granulation tissue often appears as a darker colour and may be more fragile, with a tendency to bleed more easily.

The white cell count may be increased, although the inflammatory response to surgery may appear as an initial rise in white cell count, which should settle in the first 48 hours. Levels that remain elevated may be indicative of infection, but they need to be reviewed in conjunction with other interventions. Therefore, a rising white cell count may be more indicative than just a raised white cell count, and may relate to infection occurring at invasive lines (central venous pressure [CVP] being the most common cause of infection in the critical care area).

It is not possible to ascertain from a wound swab alone whether a wound is infected. A number of practical problems exist and there is still debate about the correct way to take a swab. Common practice in most clinical areas is to take a single swab and place it in the tube provided. If the swab is delayed in getting to the laboratory, some organisms, especially the anaerobes, may die before the swab is processed.

A number of risk factors in wound infections have been identified, over several studies, and these factors can be categorised into preoperative, intraoperative and postoperative (Table 9.2)

These risk factors have been debated robustly in the literature with claims and counterclaims. Asensio Vegas et al. (1993) claim, however, that when no risk factors are present no surgical wound infections are observed, and that the rate in incidence of surgical wound infections increases from 2.5% when one risk factor is present to 53.8% when four or more risk factors are present.

Table 9.2 Risk factors associated with wound infections

Category	Risk factor
Preoperative	Smoking
	Diabetes
	COAD
	Preoperative ICU stay
	Obesity
	Advanced age (> 70 years)
	Impaired immune response
Intraoperative	Bilateral IMA
	Single IMA
	Long operation time (> 4 hours)
	Re-exploration for bleeding
	Long bypass time (> 2 hours)
Postoperative	Hypertension/hypotension
	Ventilatory support (> 48 hours)
	Inotropes
	Postoperative CPR
	Hypoxaemia
	Blood transfusion

COAD, chronic obstructive airway disease; CPR, cardiopulmonary resuscitation; ICU, intensive care unit; IMA, internal mammary artery.

Preoperative

Nicotine delays primary wound healing, but there is debate about the definition of current cigarette smoking and active smoking, and how these affect the connection. After nicotine use, wound oxygenation is decreased by microvascular obstruction as a result of platelet aggregation and a significant amount of non-functional haemoglobin.

The contribution of diabetes to wound infection is controversial as a result of a combination of contributing factors. An increased glucose level in the immediate postoperative period (48 hours) is linked to an increased risk. Increased glucose levels may be observed in non-diabetic patients if high-dose adrenaline (epinephrine) infusions are in progress or the patient is receiving total parenteral nutrition

Chronic obstructive pulmonary disease results in compromised airway clearance, predisposing to colonisation of the tracheobronchial tree. Prolonged mechanical ventilation is generally required. These patients may be more at risk of hypoxia.

The incidence of hospital-acquired infection for any hospitalised patient is widely published. It therefore follows that, if a patient requires a prolonged preoperative hospital stay, a patient's skin may become colonised with bacteria to which the patient has no resistance. The most common colonisation is with methicillin-resistant *Staphyloccus aureus* (MRSA). More patients are being screened for this occurrence so appropriate treatment can be given. The use of Hibiscrub showers is thought to counter the risk. However, the length of preoperative stay is connected to the severity of the illness and co-morbid conditions requiring inpatient management before surgery.

Obesity is defined by the use of the body mass index, defined as weight in kilograms divided by height in metres squared. Moulton (1996) suggested that, although obesity could be linked to superficial wound complications and atrial dysrhythmias, it did not predispose to deep sternal wound infection. Obese patients are particularly likely to have prolonged healing. Adipose tissue is not as well perfused as muscle, so it is reasonable to expect a greater risk of impaired wound healing as a result of tissue hypoxia. In obese individuals, the depth of the wound is greater and more dissection is required to harvest the saphenous vein, so optimal tissue oxygenation is essential.

With increasing age, there is a decreased immune response, increased risk of concurrent disease and less physiological response. Patients aged over 66 years are six times more likely to have a postoperative infection than patients up to the age of 14. Males are also more likely to develop infection because hair harbours bacteria.

Impaired immune response inhibits wound healing by interfering with the inflammatory response and reducing collagen synthesis.

Intraoperative

The use of internal mammary artery (IMA) grafts seems to be one of the most important factors relating to sternal wound complications. Diverting blood flow away from the chest wall can cause numbness and delay healing. It is advised that patients with diabetes who require revascularisation are not exposed to bilateral IMA grafts.

An open chest allows an opportunity for organisms to access the chest incision. Wound cells are damaged by drying and exposure to air and retractors. Longer procedures are more likely to be associated with blood loss and shock, reducing the general resistance of patients. Bleeding causes haematoma formation in the mediastinum, which creates an ideal medium for bacterial growth. Re-exploration further lengthens the time that internal tissues are exposed to airborne pathogens and further tissue trauma increases the risk of infection.

Cardiopulmonary bypass has a deleterious effect on the immune system, destroying phagocytes. It alters blood and blood clotting factors, providing an ideal medium for bacterial invasion and growth.

Postoperative

Postoperative care involves a very small risk of introducing bacteria into the wound. This is attributed to the fact that skin edges in direct apposition seal within a few hours, but some factors may disrupt healing.

If the patient endures prolonged or frequent periods of hypotension, perfusion pressure is diminished to the tissues, inhibiting wound healing. Ventilatory support continuing after 48 hours of surgery increases the likelihood of sternal wound infections by 9.5 times. The increased length of ventilation exposes the patient to risk factors in the intensive care environment. In addition, patients with copious amounts of sputum, which is expelled at force, are at risk of contaminating an uncovered sternal wound. Patients requiring a tracheostomy, to facilitate weaning from mechanical ventilation when secretions may appear from around the stoma, are at high risk of wound infection. In these instances, a transparent dressing is often applied at the top of the sternal wound to prevent respiratory secretions contaminating it.

The need for inotropes has the effect of shunting blood flow to vital organs at the expense of the skin and sternum (adrenaline and noradrenaline are the worst offenders). The need for inotropes alone may suggest a prolonged stay in an intensive care unit as a result of haemodynamic stability.

The need for chest compressions can cause sternal instability, and this will increase the risk of dehiscence and infection.

Low cardiac output syndrome (hypoxaemia) decreases tissue perfusion, which contributes to infection. Oxygen delivery to the wound is decreased at any given oxygen saturation during the immediate postoperative period, which is intensified in hypoxaemia.

Banked blood transfusion causes suppression of humoral immunity, which is responsible for fighting bacterial infections. Each unit transfused increases the probability of a sternal wound infection 1.05 times. There is, however, no scientific basis for withholding necessary blood products from surgical patients to try to reduce the incidence of infection.

Malnutrition is also related to infection. It has not yet been identified as an independent risk factor in the development of wound infection, but it may emphasise other risk factors, e.g. age.

Methicillin-resistant *Staphylococcus aureus*

Methicillin-resistant *Staphylococcus aureus* is an opportunistic agent, which infects patients by several modes of transmission and spreads relentlessly among those who are ill and who have received antibiotics previously. It has been a cause of hospital-acquired infection since the early 1960s. Some patients may present as a greater risk of spreading MRSA to others: MRSA isolated in sputum in patients with a productive cough, MRSA isolated from large exudating wounds where the exudate cannot be contained by dressings, and MRSA isolated from patients with exfoliative skin conditions. These patients, when possible, should be nursed in side rooms. Wherever the patient is nursed, basic infection control measures are required to reduce the spread of MRSA, as highlighted in Table 9.3.

For the most part, *Staphylococcus aureus* is a normal human commensal. It is present on the skin of about 30% of people. The bacteria are shed from the skin of carriers and become trapped in clothes. Infection may occur via the airborne route as well as through direct contact. Patients may become infected by bacteria that have been living harmlessly on

Table 9.3 Basic infection control measures to reduce the spread of infection of methicillin-resistant Staphylococcus aureus (MRSA)

- Alert organism surveillance
- Good handwashing practices to include the use of alcohol hand rub
- Appropriate decontamination of equipment between patients
- Use of gloves and aprons with body fluids, lesions and contaminated equipment
- Risk assessment and isolation of patients who are at greatest risk of spreading infection to others
- Correct handling of linen and waste
- Minimising patient movement between wards
- Avoiding overcrowding of patients
- Maintaining adequate and appropriately skill staff
- High standard of aseptic technique
- Rational use of antibiotics
- Admission screening on patients admitted from other wards, hospitals and nursing homes who are expected to be inpatients for > 48 hours
- Admission screening of patients previously colonised with MRSA

their own skin. The pathogen is carried in the nares of 20–30% of healthy humans and there is a definite connection of infection with preoperative nares carriage. Some centres have advocated routine use of a topical ointment preoperatively, regardless of carrier status.

Pressure sore development

During a period of bedrest, the patient needs to be re-positioned once haemodynamically stable, to ensure comfort, prevention of pressure sores and prevention of chest infection caused by atelectasis. The optimal position is not clearly defined. Elevating the patient's head by 30° prevents facial oedema, but the semi-recumbent or upright position is chosen to assist with respiratory problems. Positioning on to the right lateral could impede venous return, with a subsequent reduction in CVP and blood pressure. The left lateral position may diminish cardiac output with a subsequent drop in PaO_2 (Banasik and Emerson, 1996). The known benefits of lateral lying, however, outweigh the potential risks of positioning.

The development of pressure sores is associated with negative patient outcomes. After cardiac surgery patients are prone to pressure sores, with the risk increasing with corresponding haemodynamic instability, prolonged time in the operating room and neurological complications. Risk assessment involves professional judgement, complemented by the use of a pressure sore risk calculator. Risk scores have been used for several decades, the most commonly used being those of Norton (1989) and Waterlow (1991); these are usually adapted to local needs. As no risk assessment scale has yet been developed with a predictive validity and specificity (able to identify people who will not develop a sore as well as those who will), any scale must be used with and not replace clinical judgement. Its function as a memory aid must be coupled with appropriate care to deal with the risk factors identified, so reducing risk where possible.

Prevention of pressure sore development is the domain of nursing staff. This involves the promotion of patient care that prevents physical, psychological and social deterioration of the patient's current health status.

The development of a pressure sore is a product of time and pressure in combination with a number of predisposing intrinsic and extrinsic factors. There is evidence suggesting that a pressure sore develops between 1 and 5 days after pressure is applied to the skin, with a severity depending on the force and duration of the applied pressure. It is therefore vital that at least the factor of time or pressure is reduced or eliminated. Pressure becomes a problem when an individual is not able to change position independently, or is unable to feel discomfort because of neurological deficit or sedation.

The factors of time and pressure can be effectively influenced by turning the patient regularly on to one side for a short time, or nursing the patient for a longer time on alternate sides, and/or by using special pressure-relieving mattresses. Most nursing texts recommend that patients are turned/repositioned 2-hourly. There is no recognised reason why 2 hours is the crucial time. One common myth was described by Clark (1998), who states that this frequency derived from the Crimean War, where 2 hours represented the time taken for Florence Nightingale and her colleagues to visit and reposition every injured soldier on the ward. Although the origin of 2-hourly turns may not be apparent, how the patient should be repositioned has been given attention. It seems to be well established that a roll of the patient by 20–30°, with the tilt being supported by pillows, is sufficient (Defloor, 1997). The adoption of this tilted position reduces contact pressure when compared with the conventional supine position, while preventing the reduction in the supply of oxygen to vulnerable anatomical locations.

The influence of intrinsic and extrinsic factors on pressure sore development can be calculated with pressure sore risk calculators. If the extrinsic factors that cause pressure sores are eliminated, and the intrinsic factors that increase the risk of tissue damage are corrected, pressure sores can be avoided. If pressure damage does occur, which is sometimes the case despite all possible measures taken, the degree of pressure damage must be accurately recorded to ensure that appropriate care is initiated. The Stirling Pressure Sore Severity Scale (SPSSS) is a scale that attempts to introduce uniformity in the classification of pressure damage (Reid and Morison, 1994).

Eye care

Eye complications relating to mechanical ventilation are similar to the ones experienced by unconscious patients when the blink reflex may be lost, i.e. exposure risks, drying, infection and, in addition, conjunctival oedema. The last is exacerbated by the increase in venous pressure associated with intermittent positive pressure ventilation. For most patients the short period ventilated does not require intervention, but longer-term ventilated and sedated patients will require accurate assessment to determine whether the use of an artificial lubricant is required. It is important to assist the patient to close the eyelids to prevent the cornea being exposed to dust. The development of conjunctival oedema is worsened by constrictive tapes securing endotracheal (ET) tubes. Jugular venous drainage should be encouraged by head elevation. When ET suction is performed, care must be taken that air from the ventilator is not directed at the eyes.

Blurred vision is a frequently mentioned irritation to patients for several weeks after discharge.

Deep venous thrombosis

Venous thromboembolic disease contributes to morbidity and mortality after surgery in some hospitalised patients. In 1991, the *Journal of the Royal Society of Medicine* estimated that some 27 000 people die unnecessarily in hospital each year from pulmonary embolism and, in 1996, it was estimated that deep venous thrombosis (DVT) was responsible for 10% of hospital deaths annually (Office of Health Economics, 1996). It is felt that 22 000 of these deaths could be avoided by preventing the formation of blood clots in the leg. It is thought that the heparin used for cardiopulmonary bypass provides a protective function, but DVT is a recognised if not frequent complication. Practice varies between institutions in relation to the prevention of such a complication. Some hospitals make it standard practice to use preventive measures for the management of DVT, whereas most leave it to individual doctors to decide whether to use preventive measures or to rely on crisis management (i.e. diagnosis and attempted cure if symptoms are spotted). There is evidence to support preventive management being far better than crisis management.

The pathogenesis of venous thromboembolic disease was delineated over 100 years ago by Virchow, who proposed the now famous triad of stasis of the blood, vessel wall injury and hypercoagulability as the primary predisposing factors.

Venous stasis

The precise pathogenesis of stasis thrombosis is uncertain. The cul de sac behind a valve cusp in the vein is a classic area of static flow. It is thought that the low partial pressure of oxygen in this area may result in hypoxic damage to the endothelium of the valve cusp. This could result in local activation of platelets to serve as a nucleus for thrombus formation. This stasis may be enhanced by prolonged periods of bedrest.

Vessel injury

The vessel endothelium plays an important role in thromboresistance, serving as a barrier between the blood and the thrombogenic substances in the subendothelium tissues. Vessel injury may occur when the saphenous veins are used in bypass grafting.

Hypercoagulability

Certain hereditary and acquired coagulation abnormalities predispose some people to thrombolic disease. Postoperatively, numerous alterations in platelets, coagulation proteins and fibrinolytic activity have been identified which could predispose to thrombus.

Although the components of Virchow's triad are often discussed separately, they are interwoven. One component may predominate, but their combined effect ultimately leads to the development of venous thrombosis. A symptomatic calf vein thrombosis may lead to subsequent pulmonary embolism (PE), but it is generally felt that the thrombus arising in the calf must extend to the popliteal vein or beyond before there is a significant risk of embolisation.

Several risk factors have been identified in relation to DVT (Table 9.4). It is suggested that 50% of all DVTs begin on the operating table and 75% will be present within 48 hours of surgery (O'Meara and Kaufman, 1990). The risk of DVT development during surgery is present in any operation requiring a general anaesthesia of more than 30 min. Obesity increases intra-abdominal pressure and interferes with venous return, and poses a greater risk of development of DVT than for the non-obese patient.

There is a strong relationship between increasing age and DVT development, the risk increasing significantly after the age of 50 years. With advancing age, the soleal veins become tortuous and calf muscle mass decreases. Both these changes reduce the efficiency of the venous pump and contribute to a decrease in the rate of venous return. Diseases and situations that cause paralysis or immobilise the lower limbs are associated with a high incidence of DVT. People confined to a bed or restricted to sitting for long periods are associated with greater risk. The calf muscle pump is the main source of venous return, forcing blood towards the heart. Reduced movement of the calf muscle leads to a reduction in venous return. Immobility causes venous stasis. The incidence of venous thrombosis is increased for patients with cardiac disease, particularly those with congestive heart failure.

Table 9.4 Risk factors in the development of venous thromboembolism

Category	Example
Congenital	Antithrombin III deficiency or dysfunction
	Protein C deficiency
	Protein S deficiency
	Dysfibrinogenaemia
	Plasminogen deficiency
	Plasminogen activator dysfunction
	Heparin cofactor II deficiency
	Homocystinuria
Surgical	General anaesthesia
	Postoperative:
	• orthopaedic surgery
	• urological surgery
	• colon surgery
	Multiple trauma
Gynaecology and obstetrics	Pelvic surgery
	Radiotherapy for uterine cancer
	Pregnancy and puerperium
Miscellaneous	Previous thromboembolic disease
	Varicose veins
	Age
	Obesity

Symptoms

Only 3.5% of patients who develop DVT will have clinical symptoms (Caprini and Natonson, 1991), which include a swollen and painful calf or thigh, palpable vein cords in the calf or thigh, increase in skin temperature over the thrombosis, and local skin discoloration secondary to cyanosis. As the clinical signs can be vague, an individual with a suspected DVT will usually be referred to radiology. Procedures confirming diagnosis can be invasive or non-invasive. The most frequently used invasive test is the venogram, which involves the injection of radio-opaque dye into a distal dorsal foot vein before taking radiographic films to identify whether a thrombus is present. Doppler ultrasonography is a non-invasive, less expensive test that is quicker than a venogram. It can be used to detect calf vein or proximal vein thrombosis, but is less sensitive at detecting calf thrombosis.

Prophylactic methods are aimed at combating the factors implicated in the aetiology of thrombosis: hypercoagulability (pharmacological methods); vascular stasis (mechanical methods); and damage to the vessel wall. Surgeons may choose a combination or single methods of prevention, based on preference and experience, although others will introduce methods based on assessment of risk. The greater the risk the greater the intervention (Table 9.5 shows risk categories).

Table 9.5 Categorising risk of deep venous thrombosis

Low risk
10% risk of developing calf vein thrombosis, one risk factor present
Age < 40
No additional risk factors
Minor surgery < 30 minutes
Uncomplicated medical patients bed bound for less than 24 h
Pregnancy

Moderate risk
10–40% risk of calf vein thrombosis, two to four risk factors
Age < 40 years with history of fracture or thrombosis
Age > 40 years
Surgery > 30 minutes
Malignancy, 40–60 years
Trauma, no fracture
Uncomplicated myocardial infarction
Pregnancy with varicose veins or history of thrombosis

High risk
40–80% risk of calf vein thrombosis, more than four risk factors
Age 40–60 with history of thrombosis or fracture
Extensive general surgery
Joint replacement
Malignancy over age 60
Major trauma with fracture
Complex medical history

Ambulation

The simplest method of prophylaxis is early mobilisation. Walking contracts the leg muscles, stimulating the venous pump and eliminating stasis. It is extremely effective in low-risk patients (Table 9.5), but it will be effective only if it minimally consists of 5 min of walking each hour.

If early mobilisation is not possible, graduated compression stockings may be warranted. These are known to be beneficial in low-risk surgical patients (Goucke, 1989), but their efficacy in preventing DVT in moderate- and high-risk patients is uncertain. The external compression of anti-embolism stockings applies a controlled pressure to the skin to help reduce oedema, usually present after surgery, as a result of both vein harvesting and a positive fluid balance after cardiopulmonary bypass, and this aids venous return. In addition, if the amount of external pressure is graduated so that it is higher at the ankle and lower at the knee, blood velocity within the deep venous system is increased, counteracting any venous insufficiency.

Stockings appear to be a benign therapy, but stockings that are too tight can cause complications, e.g. peroneal nerve injury when the fabric bunches behind the knee. Anti-embolism stockings should be fitted only after a detailed patient assessment. A stocking that fits correctly will produce an effective graduation in pressure and will be comfortable to wear without forming tight bands at the knee. The leg(s) should be measured early in the morning or immediately after removal of stockings to minimise the effect of oedema. Measurement should be taken daily with the patient's feet flat on the floor, and both legs should be measured to identify variation between the limbs. The actual measurements required are dependent on whether thigh-length or knee-length stockings are in use and on the manufacturer.

Thigh-length versus knee-length stockings

There is debate about the differences in the complication rate using knee-length as opposed to thigh-length stockings. Some studies suggest that there is no difference and that it should be led by patient comfort. It is suggested that clots forming in the femoral region usually have more devastating effects, but the pressure exerted to the veins above the knee is minimal despite the use of stockings. If stockings are used to provide support to the limb from which vein harvest has occurred, this should possibly dictate the length of stockings, e.g. wound to the knee or thigh. Patients who have had coronary artery bypass grafts using the vein/artery of an arm should have an elastic bandage applied to the full length of the arm. The arm must not be used for venepuncture, cannulation or monitoring blood pressure for 3 months after surgery.

Heparin

Heparin is the most widely used drug in the prophylaxis of DVT. The common dosage of low-dose heparin (LDH) is 5000 units subcutaneously 2 hours before surgery and continued until the patient is fully mobile. Schedules of 8- and 12-hour dosing have both been found to be effective (Goucke, 1989). If the patient is to go on bypass, the preoperative heparin is usually omitted and, as a result of the subsequent heparinisation, it is not recommenced for 24 hours. To administer LDH, the injection should ideally be given in the lower abdomen, deep in the subcutaneous fat. The injection site should not be massaged after administration and the abdominal site should be rotated. Routine monitoring of partial thromboplastin time is not required. Low-molecular-weight heparin is thought to provoke fewer bleeding complications, and administration is the same as for LDH.

Mobilisation

Early ambulation is possible and very beneficial for most patients, but the degree of mobilisation postoperatively is dependent on the individual patient. Suitable patients should try climbing stairs (which would be most patients), and very few patients need to have their bed brought downstairs on discharge. Toilets are very often upstairs and most patients would be able to walk upstairs freely before discharge. Patients who are able to climb stairs demonstrate an acceptable level of ambulation and it may be a deciding factor for discontinuing subcutaneous heparin.

When patients are taken to try the stairs, it is worth remembering that they will probably not have a long walk before going upstairs at home. Therefore a wheelchair to a flight of stairs is acceptable, particularly for patients who have a physical restriction to mobilisation or for a dyspnoeic patient. It is not advisable for patients to attempt the stairs after a meal or exertion. Patients who live in a bungalow should be assessed individually as to whether they are required to complete the stairs before discharge. Patients who live in bungalows should not automatically complete the stairs before discharge.

For patients who require prolonged periods of bedrest, the joints should be positioned to follow natural anatomical flexion. Lack of limb movement may lead to tendon shortening and stiffness with subsequent deformity and pain, e.g. drop foot. This may be avoided by effective joint positioning, adequate use of active exercises and the use of splints. This care must be complemented with minimisation of physiological stress by ensuring that the patient receives adequate nutrition to prevent muscle wasting (Ashurst, 1997).

References

Ashurst S (1997) Nursing care of the mechanically ventilated patient in ITU (1). *Br J Nursing* 6: 447–54.
Asensio Vegas A, Monge Jodra V, Soriano C, Lopez R, Gil A, Lizon Garcia M (1993) Surgical wound infection: the risk factors and predictive model. *Med Clin (Barc)* 100: 521–5.
Banasik J, Emerson R (1996) Effect of lateral position on arterial and venous blood gases in post operative cardiac surgical patients. *Am J Crit Care* 5: 121–6.
Caprini JA, Natonson RA (1989) Post-operative deep vein thrombosis: current clinical considerations. *Semin Thromb Haemost* 15: 244–9.
Clark M (1998) Repositioning to prevent pressure sores – what is the evidence *Nursing Standard* 13(3): 58–64
Defloor T (1997) The effect of posture and mattress on the development of pressure ulcers. In: *7th European Conference on Advances in Wound Management.* London: Macmillan Magazines.
Goucke CR (1989) Prophylaxis against venous thromboembolism. *Anaesth Intensive Care* 17: 458–65.
Hussey LC, Leeper B, Hynan C (1998) Development of the sternal wound infection prediction scale. *Heart Lung* 27: 326–36.
Loop F, Lytle B, Cosgrove B et al. (1990) Sternal wound complications after isolated coronary artery bypass grafting: early and late mortality: morbidity and cost of care. *Ann Thorac Surg* 49: 179–87.
Moulton M (1996) Obesity is not a risk factor for significant adverse outcomes. *Circulation* 94(suppl 9): 1187–92.
Norton D (1989) Calculating the risk: reflections on the Norton Scale. *Decubitus* 2(3): 24–31.
Office of Health Economics (1996) *Deep Vein Thrombosis and Pulmonary Embolism.* London: OHE.
O'Meara PM, Kaufman EE (1990) Prophylaxis for venous thromboembolism in total hip arthroplasty: a review. *Orthopedics* 13: 173–8.
Reid J, Morison M (1994) Towards a consensus, classification of pressure sores. *J Wound Care* 3: 157–60.
Sarr MG, Gott VL, Townsend R (1984) Mediastinal infection after cardiac surgery. *Ann Thorac Surg* 38: 415–23.
Sellick J, Stelmach M, Mylotte J (1991) Surveillance of surgical wound infections following open heart surgery. *Infect Control Hosp Epidemiol* 12: 591–6.
Ulicny K, Hiratzha L, Williams R et al. (1990) Sternotomy infection: poor prediction by acute phase response and delayed hypersensitivity. *Ann Thorac Surg* 50: 949–58.
Waterlow J (1991) A policy that protects the Waterlow Score Prevention/Treatment Policy. *Professional Nurse* 6: 258–62.
Weintraub WS, Jones EL, Craver J, Cohen C (1989) Determinants of prolonged length of hospital stay after coronary bypass. *Circulation* 8: 276–84.
Wipke-Jervis D, Stotts N, Skov M, Carrieri-Kohlman C (1996) Frequency, manifestations and correlates of impaired healing of saphenous vein harvest incisions. *Heart Lung* 25: 108–16.

CHAPTER 10

Psychological care

A common complication that has been recognised after cardiac surgery is behavioural disturbance. This condition has been referred to under many headings, the most common of which are postcardiotomy delirium or 'pump syndrome'. The reason for the disturbance is unclear, but the syndrome is thought to occur in 7–72% of patients depending on the defining characteristics (Heller, 1979; Sadler, 1981; Farrimond, 1984; Briggs, 1991). Symptoms may include fatigue, distraction, confusion, disorientation, restlessness, clouding of consciousness, incoherence, fear, anxiety, excitement, illusions, hallucinations and delusions (Blachy and Starr, 1964; Briggs, 1991; Crippen and Erimakov, 1992).

Whatever the symptoms, these patients offer a challenge to nursing staff. Patients developing the syndrome fall into two categories: hyper-active–hyperalert and hypoactive–hypoalert. Patients in the hyperactive–hyperalert group frequently seem intent on removing every piece of equipment and line necessary for treatment while simultaneously attempting to climb over cot sides. They are usually agitated and can become aggressive, presenting as a danger not only to themselves but also to staff.

The second group of patients (hypoactive–hypoalert) are passive and drowsy and may easily be overlooked. These patients often experience vivid dreams and hallucinations, and may appear to be vacant or just stare into space. The condition is usually identified only through inappropriate words or by the patient 'being out of character', as perceived by relatives. Although patients in either group do not seem to remember this stage of their recovery, a large number (10–30%) continue to experience vivid dreams or hallucinations for several months after cardiac surgery.

Symptoms usually present 48 hours after surgery, but may be delayed if the patient has undergone a prolonged period of sedation and ventilation. The major disturbance usually lasts for no more than 72 hours during which time care should be given to promote the patient's general recovery and prevent the patient endangering his or her recovery.

Over the years, several theories have been formulated with regard to the reason for the behavioural disturbances, and these theories can also be linked to the development of nursing and medicine. The causes are summarised in Table 10.1. In the late 1950s and during the 1960s, it was noted that patients undergoing cardiac surgery displayed some changes in their behaviour, which were generally unrecognised in general surgical patients. With medicine dominating the care, physical/physiological reasons were sought, and those forwarded related to the condition of individual patients preoperatively, intraoperatively and postoperatively (Farrimond, 1984). Observation of patients suggested that behavioural disturbances were more likely to occur in older patients, and those who had a sicker preoperative course. The age of the patient is no longer that significant because surgery is performed on older patients than in the 1960s. Patients with long-standing atrial fibrillation were considered a high risk, and it has now been proved that patients with atrial fibrillation are more at risk of neurological deficits in general, not just as a result of surgery.

Table 10.1 Influential factors in the development of the 'pump syndrome'

Decade	Influencing factor	Examples
1960s	Physiological	Age Preoperative condition Atrial fibrillation Bypass time Hypoxia Temperature Biochemistry
1970s	Environmental factors	Sleep Noise Separation Communication Immobilisation
1980s	Psychological	Social class Anxiety types
1990s	Multi-factorial	Individual differences

Much of the blame was also directed at the cardiopulmonary bypass, hence the term 'postcardiotomy delirium' or 'pump syndrome'. It was thought that the longer the time spent on the cardiopulmonary bypass, the greater the risk of behavioural disturbances. It is now recognised that, the longer the patient is on bypass, the more complications he or she is likely to experience, but patients have also displayed the manifestations of 'pump syndrome' after surgery for which cardiopulmonary bypass was not required. The frequency of behavioural disturbances has also reduced since the introduction of filters in the arterial line from the pump oxygenator to the patient.

Postoperatively, a number of factors were seen to be influential. Hypoxia was a popular reason, and this has been identified as an isolated cause of confusion and agitation in all hospitalised patients. Patients are usually well oxygenated during surgery, but postoperatively, during a period of ventilation or later, they may experience a degree of hypoxia and this would account for the onset of symptoms 24 hours after surgery. It is suggested that, at any one time, 10–15% of hospitalised patients may display signs of confusion. A large variation in core temperature postoperatively was also considered important. Patients who experience temperature swings, or demonstrate a hyperpyrexia immediately postoperatively with a sudden return to apyrexia, are seen as most at risk and now attention is given to ensuring that, when the patient becomes normothermic centrally, aggressive re-warming methods are discontinued. Disturbances in biochemistry are also relevant. It is now apparent that several patients experience a degree of renal failure postoperatively, and this could cause an alteration in mental functioning.

By the end of the 1960s, despite identifying the factors mentioned, and implementing care to reduce the factors, behavioural disturbances were still seen. It had also became apparent that other patients nursed in an intensive care setting were also displaying behavioural disturbances, and at this time attention switched from the physiological factors to environmental factors. The behavioural disturbances were termed 'ICU psychosis' (Briggs, 1991). The most important environmental factors identified were sleep deprivation, noise, separation, communication and immobilisation (Tucker, 1993).

It has long been established that sleep is an important part of the healing process and that more sleep than usual is required when an individual is ill and in hospital. Patients who can recall their experiences in intensive care, for example, report problems encountered with sleep, and sleep deprivation remains problematic. Much of the routine nursing care is performed on an hourly or 2-hourly basis, although it is believed that, for a patient to gain any benefit from sleep, the patient must complete a full 90-minute cycle. Further studies (S Close, 1988, unpublished study) suggest that in a postoperative night a patient is disturbed on average 100 times for nursing procedures, e.g. observations. Attention is therefore paid to the frequency as well as the need for interventions.

Sleep can be promoted by encouraging the normal sleep–wake cycle. Although it may not be possible to access natural daylight, the normal day–night cycle can be simulated by adjusting lighting as well as noise. Pain perception is greatest at night and, if inadequate analgesia is given, a vicious cycle of increased pain and reduced sleep develops. Inappropriate intervention to relieve pain and discomfort can exacerbate the patient's feelings of fear and anxiety.

During a period of hospitalisation, particularly within intensive care, a patient is bombarded with strange and unfamiliar noises. The International Noise Council recommends that the volume of noise in the intensive care should be no more than 45 decibels (dB) during the day and 20 dB at night, but the noise actually averages from 50 dB to 70 dB consistently. Much of the noise is that generated by equipment, although this can be reduced slightly by the appropriate setting of monitor and ventilator alarms.

During a period of hospitalisation, particularly in intensive care, patients are removed from their familiar surroundings and the company of familiar people, which highlights the value of preoperative visits to the intensive care area which allows patients to gain some familiarisation with an area and staff. Allowing a policy of open visiting to this area may alleviate some of this stressor (McHaffie, 1992). Billings (1990) demonstrated that limiting access to relatives increased patient anxiety.

Most patients lose the ability to communicate after cardiac surgery as a result of the presence of an ET tube or the use of sedation. Effective communication is, however, seen as a key strategy in the prevention of behavioural disturbances. All patients should receive explanations about care activities, about their condition and any additional information that will contribute to their orientation. An important problem is that unresponsiveness is mistaken for unconsciousness, so all patients should be treated as if they are conscious and able to communicate. A large proportion of patients who are awake may have problems with communication as a result of the presence of an ET tube or tracheostomy. Despite many aids being available to assist with communication, the problem may remain and the patient can become frustrated.

The use of invasive techniques and therapies required after surgery can result in the patient experiencing a feeling of being tied down. The resultant immobilisation will exaggerate sensations of fear, anxiety and helplessness. Patients who are able to recall being intubated describe the presence of the ET tube as being incredibly uncomfortable, particularly where they were being moved or turned when the nurses were not concentrating on supporting the patient's head. An oral tube may provide a constant gagging feeling. Several patients mention that they make attempts to support their tube in the 'optimum position' only to have a nurse grab their hand or shout for them to stop it.

Behavioural disturbances do not occur only in patients admitted to intensive care; indeed, they can occur in patients admitted to any area of the hospital, and similarly not all patients admitted to intensive care experience behavioural disturbances. In the 1980s, concentration moved away from environmental factors to psychological variations, namely social class and anxiety types (Farrimond, 1984). Heller (1979) attempted to identify personality types by performing psychological tests of personality, but the studies were not conclusive (Dubin, 1979). These studies did, however, show differing rates of incidence depending on the social class of the patient. Members of higher social classes, e.g. doctors, teachers and lawyers, tended to display a higher incidence than lower social classes, e.g. factory workers and miners (Sadler, 1981). It is thought that this is a result of higher social class members becoming dependent on others when they are usually independent and in charge of their lives.

Janis (1971) classified the degree of anxiety displayed by patients into three categories: high anxiety, moderate anxiety and low anxiety. Patients in the high-anxiety groups are thought to express vulnerability, are unable to sleep and have negative thoughts regarding the operation and their future. Postoperatively, these patients remain anxious and concerned about their future. A small percentage of patients in this group may require professional counselling postoperatively.

Patients experiencing little or no anxiety deny feeling worried; indeed, they trivialise the operation or deny any illness. Generally they sleep well, but they do not want to know about the treatment in an effort to shield themselves from reality (McHaffie, 1992). Postoperatively, they display anxiety through anger and resentment towards staff. Both these groups are likely to develop postcardiotomy delirium.

In contrast, the patients in the moderate-anxiety category tend to ask questions and communicate their anxiety over certain aspects of their treatment (e.g. pain, anaesthetic). This suggests that a degree of anxiety can be beneficial, but it is a fine balance and can easily become detrimental. Anxiety levels therefore range from those that can alert, arouse and motivate to those that can result in paralysing panic. Table 10.2 illustrates the main reasons for anxiety in patients undergoing cardiac surgery. In 1977, Layne and Yudofsky demonstrated that nursing interventions can adjust the amount of anxiety expressed and preadmission clinics are just a small example of an intervention that can increase communication and decrease the amount of anxiety experienced.

In the 1990s there seems to be agreement that no one factor can be identified as an indicator of 'pump syndrome', and optimum care should be given to minimise physiological changes and environmental stressors and relieve anxiety, in the hope that there is a reduced incidence of behavioural disturbances.

As a consequence, the causes of postcardiotomy delirium are currently considered to be multifactorial (Crippen and Erimakov, 1992).

Table 10.2 Identified causes of anxiety in the patient undergoing cardiac surgery

Cause	Contributing factor
Hospitalisation	Previous experience
	Fear of unknown
	Media coverage
Surgery	Anaesthetic
	Anticipation of pain
	Threat to life (Davenport, 1991)
	Discussion of mortality (Cheetham, 1993)
Family	Anxiety of family (Roberts, 1991)

Care of the family/relatives

Cardiac surgery poses a great strain on the patient's family, especially the spouse or partner. The early postoperative period may be threatening because of the nature of the surgery, the risk of complications and separation from their loved ones, as well as feeling uncomfortable in the intensive care unit with all its crowded facilities. Families have identified that the time spent waiting while the patient is in surgery is the worst part of the hospital experience, during which time the spouse/family has little contact with the health-care professional. They are commonly most anxious to know if any complications have occurred during surgery.

The most important need of the spouse/family in the early postoperative period is provision of information. Such provision of information helps the family to cope with the stressful situation. The patient is often returned from a critical care area within 24 hours of surgery. This transfer may be viewed as threatening, because the nurse: patient ratio decreases dramatically. Specific questions may be asked despite the relevant information being shared preoperatively, and this demonstrates an inability to retain information during the stressful preoperative period. It is also important to member that an anxious relative increases the anxiety of a patient (Rayleigh, 1990).

Learning needs generally occur at an earlier time during the recovery period for spouses/partners than they do for patients. This is because the patient has a combination of fatigue, incisional and musculoskeletal discomfort, postoperative depression and opioid analgesia, all affecting the readiness to learn, returning to work and sexual relationships.

Despite the advances in technology and the introduction of new drugs, there remains a recognised risk of mortality after cardiac surgery, the risk varying between patients according to individualised risk factors. It is also inevitable that some patients die in the immediate postoperative period, in the operating room or in the recovery area, or after a period of stability and recovery. All patients and significant others should be informed of the mortality risk and this could open up communication about this issue. Many patients treat this information in a positive manner, identifying that the chances of success are greater than the risk of failure, whereas some are more negative in the receipt of this information and focus on the mortality rate, when it may be as low as 1–2%.

For some patients, death may result from a cardiac arrest when resuscitation attempts fail. On other occasions, death may be over a protracted period. The patient may experience major complications resulting from multi-system failure. These patients may pose ethical dilemmas for staff and relatives. Communication between all parties is of crucial importance to ensure that all views are represented and that any decisions taken with regard to withholding (including resuscitation) or withdrawing treatment have the agreement or, at the very least, the understanding of all parties. Living wills, while providing some insight into the patient's wishes, are not valid in these instances. They are only legally valid in terminal illness where there is a predicted course, whereas, in these instances, there is not a predicted course.

Debate has focused on whether relatives should be present at resuscitation attempts or when treatment is withdrawn. The issue cannot be generalised and must be assessed on an individual basis. A similar debate arises surrounding whether, after a resuscitation attempt, equipment should be removed from around the bed area. Some relatives need to see the equipment to be certain that all attempts at resuscitation have occurred, whereas others wish to see that the patient is at rest.

References

Billings I (1990) Being a patient. *Surg Nurse* 11–12.

Blachy PH, Starr A (1964) Post cardiotomy delirium. *Am J Psychiatry* **121**: 371.

Briggs D (1991) Preventing ICU psychosis. *Nursing Times* **87**(19): 30–1.

Cheetham D (1993) Pre-operative visits by ITU nurses: recommendations for practice. *Intensive Crit Care Nursing* **9**: 253–62.

Crippen D, Erimakov S (1992) Stress, agitation and brain failure in critical care medicine. *Crit Care Nursing Q* **15**(2): 52–74.

Davenport V (1991) The waiting period prior to cardiac surgery when complicated by sudden cancellation. *Intensive Care Nursing* **7**: 105–13.

Dubin WR (1979) Post-cardiotomy delirium. A critical review. *Am J Psychiatry* **121**: 371.

Farrimond P (1984) Post cardiotomy delirium. *Nursing Times* **80**(30): 39–41.

Heller S (1979) Psychiatric complications of open heart surgery. *N Engl J Med* **283**: 1015–19.

Janis IL (1971) *Stress and Frustration*. New York: Harcourt.

Layne O, Yudofsky S (1971). In: Sadler (1981).

McHaffie HE (1992) Coping: an essential element of nursing. *J Adv Nursing* **17**: 933–40.

Raleigh EH (1990) Significant others benefit from pre-operative information. *J Adv Nursing* **15**: 941–5.

Roberts R (1991) Preventing PPD after surgery. *Nursing* **4**(27): 28–30.

Sadler P (1981) Incidence, degree and duration of post cardiotomy delirium. *Heart Lung* **10**: 1084–91.

Tucker L (1993) Post pump delirium. *Intensive Crit Care Nursing* **9**: 269–7.

Further reading

Ferguson JA (1992) Pain following coronary artery bypass grafting: an exploration of contributing factors. *Intensive Crit Care Nursing* **8**: 153–62.

CHAPTER 11

Discharge and rehabilitation

There is no agreed optimum day for discharge after cardiac surgery. Discharge routinely occurs after between 4 and 10 days for patients who have experienced an uncomplicated recovery from bypass grafts and valve replacements. Patients admitted for valve replacements usually require a longer hospital stay than bypass graft patients. Delayed discharge has implications for patient morbidity and hospital costs, e.g. the longer a hospital stay, the greater the risk of hospital-acquired infection. Psychologically it can cause depression in the patient. The complications of cardiac surgery can be divided into cardiac and non-cardiac, and it is often the latter that delays postoperative discharge. Readjustment after surgery is a long slow process, whereas the length of hospitalisation continues to shorten.

There is no 'normal' recovery time after heart operations, much depending on the preoperative physical condition, intraoperative progress and development of postoperative complications. However, most patients will take from 6 to 12 weeks to make a satisfactory recovery. Sanchez et al. (1994) suggest that day 8 postoperatively is the safest day to discharge patients because of known time-related incidents of complications, although some patients may be discharged as early as day 3. These patients may not necessarily have made a superior recovery, but the hospital may have a liaison service to follow these patients up closely at home for the next 3 days. This service is usually offered only to patients who live in close proximity to the operating hospital.

In preparation for discharge, in addition to physical care, a large proportion of nursing care includes the provision of information aimed at reducing the risks associated with the development of coronary artery disease, and to prevent potential complications associated with the surgery. The topics of exercise, diet and smoking are usually reviewed.

Patients are encouraged to exercise regularly, eat a low-fat, low-sodium or healthy diet, depending on cholesterol and sodium levels, and to stop smoking, although this education is also usually given before surgery if the patient has required hospitalisation for their treated condition. After risk reduction, care is taken to instruct the patient and spouse/partner in various aspects of recovery, including reducing the risks of complications occurring. Resuming sexual activity, returning to work, reducing stress, resuming normal daily activities, pain management and medication are generally reviewed.

The issues concerning patients are very individual. Women tend to express concerns relating to who would be the carers at home, whereas men mainly express concerns relating to physical recovery, return to work and long-term activities (Barnason et al., 2000).

Diet

Patency of vein grafts for more than 1 year after bypass may be enhanced by the control of the risk factors for arteriosclerosis. Bypass surgery has a favourable effect on symptoms and useful life expectancy in many patients, but it does not cure arteriosclerotic heart disease, and symptoms of myocardial ischaemia will return to all patients at some point. Once the patient has recovered from the operation he or she should be counselled about the importance of maintaining an appropriate body weight, caloric reduction, and optimising low blood lipid levels. Elevated lipids have been identified to be an important risk factor for the atherosclerotic disease in saphenous vein bypass grafts. Aggressive dietary and pharmacological control of the serum cholesterol have been shown to retard the progression of the vein graft atherosclerosis. For patients who have had surgery for non-atherosclerotic disease, a healthy diet is encouraged to prevent this.

Fats

There are three main kinds of fat present in our diet:

- saturated
- polyunsaturated
- monounsaturated.

If a food contains fat, it is always a mixture of these three. Currently, fat amounts to 39.1% of our total calories, but a 'Health of a Nation' target is to reduce this intake to 35%. Levels of cholesterol in the blood are influenced by dietary fat in addition to physical activity, smoking, body weight and genetics. Low-density lipoproteins (LDLs) are the main carriers of blood cholesterol; they are the main cause of atherosclerosis and are often called 'bad cholesterol'. Conversely, high-density lipoproteins (HDLs) are referred to as 'good cholesterol', because high HDL levels appear to decrease the risk of coronary heart disease.

It is hoped that the patient admitted for surgery will have had a cholesterol level taken, and the diet recommended should reflect the result. Patients with a cholesterol within normal limits should be encouraged to take a healthy diet, low-fat diets being specifically reserved for those with a high cholesterol.

Fibre

The chemical definition of dietary fibre is non-starch polysaccharide, of which there are insoluble and soluble types. Both play a part in healthy eating, but only the soluble type has a role in cardiac protection.

Insoluble polysaccharide helps prevent constipation and diverticular disease. It is present in unrefined cereal products, e.g. wholemeal bread, wholemeal pasta and wholewheat or bran breakfast cereals. Soluble non-starch polysaccharides may help lower LDL-cholesterol and blood glucose. They are present in oats, beans, fruit and vegetables.

Sodium

A high sodium intake can influence blood pressure. Salt is the most common source of sodium (as sodium chloride). In the UK, between 65% and 85% of sodium chloride comes from manufactured food. A reduced sodium diet is one that is low in processed food. The trend of simply avoiding salt at the table or using a salt substitute has little impact on total sodium if large amounts of processed foods continue to feature in the diet.

Obesity

The body mass index ($BMI = weight [kg]/height [m]^2$) defines grades of under-nutrition and obesity. Weight begins to influence coronary heart disease risk somewhere between a BMI of 25 and 30, and increases dramatically above a BMI of 30. Other risk factors are linked to obesity:

- hypercholesterolaemia
- hypertension
- poor blood glucose control in diabetes.

Reduced physical activity often plays a part in the causation of obesity. There is evidence to suggest, however, that regular physical activity, even in obese individuals, substantially improves an individual's risk. A BMI of between 20 and 25 denotes the ideal weight.

In addition to obesity, the body shape of a person can influence the risk of developing coronary heart disease. Central obesity, or the apple shape, poses a greater risk to health compared with femoral obesity (pear shape). It is possible for central obesity to occur with a healthy BMI between 20 and 25, and this still requires a weight-loss effort. A simple measurement of waist circumference – the midway point between the lowest rib and the iliac crest with the patient standing at the end of gentle expiration – can be used to indicate the risk to health. General guidelines using waist circumference are:

- There is no need to lose weight if:
  - men have a waist circumference of 94 cm or less
  - women have a waist circumference of 80 cm or less.
- Weight reduction should be advised if:
  - men have a waist circumference of 102 cm or more
  - women have a waist circumference of 88 cm or more.

Dietary advice

For a balanced diet, a variety of foods should be encouraged. Healthy eating does not mean perfect eating, but emphasis should be placed on plenty of fruit, vegetables and starchy foods in line with Mediterranean dietary habits. Patients who are obese, or have a raised cholesterol, should ideally be started on a low-fat diet. The timing of this change warrants attention. Most patients have a reduced appetite after a period of hospitalisation, and initially it is important that the patient takes a normal diet so 'diets' should not be commenced until 4 weeks after discharge.

Fruit and vegetables: five a day

A daily intake of 400 g of fruit or vegetables (equivalent to five portions) or more helps reduce the risks of heart disease or cancer. This consumption excludes potatoes and assumes that the five portions are different. It does not matter whether the fruit or vegetables are fresh, frozen, tinned or dried. However, tinned fruit in juice is recommended rather than in syrup and tinned vegetables in unsalted water.

Bread, potatoes, rice, pasta and cereals

These foods provide bulk, vitamins and minerals. They are naturally low in fat, but the food that accompanies them or the way that they are cooked can increase the fat content significantly.

Dairy foods

These provide calcium, vitamins and minerals. They can be high in fat so lower-fat versions should be encouraged.

Meat

Meat products that are high in fat and salt should be discouraged. However, meat is the best source of first-class proteins, so small amounts of lean meat or chicken without skin can be encouraged.

Fish

Fish is a useful source of protein and, in an effort to reduce the intake of red meat, with a potentially high fat content, patients should be encouraged to eat fish.

Nuts

Nuts are good sources of protein, fibre, vitamins and minerals. Most are high in fat. Unsalted nuts are acceptable as a replacement for meat or fish, but calories and fat may add up if eaten as a snack.

Fats and oils

Restricted use of all fats and oils should be advised.

If patients do not need to lose weight, but do need to reduce their intake of fat, e.g. hypercholesterolaemia, a greater intake of starchy foods to prevent unnecessary weight loss should be encouraged.

Alcohol

Epidemiological studies suggest that moderate drinkers have a lower relative risk of coronary heart disease than abstainers and those with alcohol problems. Possible explanations relate to the effects of alcohol consumption on blood lipids and lipoprotein levels, as well as the process of thrombogenesis. Excessive alcohol intake is a risk factor for heart disease. At high levels it increases the risk of cardiac arrhythmias, cardiomyopathy and sudden heart attacks. However, unlike cigarette smoking, there are levels of alcohol consumption that are considered to be beneficial to health. A report by the Department of Health (1995) concluded that there is evidence to show that, in men over 40 years and postmenopausal women, drinking 1–2 units of alcohol a day can offer protection from coronary heart disease. After surgery, alcohol can be consumed, but interactions with medication particularly warfarin require attention.

Smoking

Returning to a smoke-free environment can hasten recovery by reducing the risk of complications and increase the life expectancy of the patient. Advice on smoking, if appropriate, should be given to the patient and family members. Tobacco constituents of carbon monoxide and nicotine make the blood more likely to clot because they interfere with the formation of fibrin. It also increases the permeability of arteries to cholesterol, allowing the cholesterol levels to build up.

Management of pain

Moore (1995) discovered that, for the first 3 weeks after surgery, women tended to experience symptoms such as numbness and discomfort of the chest, whereas men reported chest incision discomfort. In addition, women are more likely to experience chest wall discomfort for a longer period postoperatively, with many still reporting chest discomfort after 18 months, although generally women are able to cope successfully with this discomfort. Among women, the younger patients are more likely to report this discomfort (Rowe and King, 1998). The difference in experience between the sexes suggests that the discomfort could arise from an anatomical relationship, the result of the tissue and nerve disruption after dissection of the internal mammary artery (IMA) from the chest wall. Stereotypically, complaints of chronic discomfort are associated with psychological states and this is now being disproved. However, women should be warned that long-term chest wall discomfort is a relatively frequent occurrence and may involve the sensation of itchiness, numbness and tenderness.

Patients should be actively encouraged to take analgesia on discharge, the type being taken dependent on what was required for pain control during hospitalisation. They should be weaned off analgesia slowly and, even when the patient feels that the pain is under control, analgesia should be used to ensure that the patient remains pain free, rather than taking it as a cure when pain is experienced. Analgesia at night and in the morning should be the minimum encouraged in the first 4 weeks. Inadequate pain control will result in other complications, such as chest infections and the results of immobilisation.

Rest and exercise

Patients appear to tire easily during the first 2 weeks, and this is the result of several things: the large dose of general anaesthetic, the disruption of normal sleep patterns, and the potential discomfort and anxiety as a result of surgery. Normal sleep patterns need to be restored, but it is important that the quest for rest does not jeopardise the need gradually to increase the amount of exercise taken. Most patients would have demonstrated an ability to exercise (walking or climbing stairs) before discharge, and patients should continue to exercise and increase the amount performed daily. When possible, patients should not have their house rearranged by bringing the bed downstairs, because climbing the stairs is a very necessary part of the recovery process.

Patients should aim to take a daily walk – a cheap and easy form of exercise. Ideally, in the initial weeks, walks should be with a companion at a pace at which a conversation can be held without dyspnoea occurring. Although it is important that the distance walked steadily increases, aiming to walk a mile a day is frequently recommended. During the initial days, the patient may experience discomfort or aches around the chest, shoulders or back. This is inevitable when muscles and bones are healing. This discomfort improves, but oral analgesics can be taken to lessen the discomfort experienced.

In poorer weather, it is not recommended that the patients walk outside, but to continue increasing activity. Climbing the stairs is a form of replacement exercise. Regular activity will help to prevent stiffness. Many centres now hold exercise sessions in a gym supervised by hospital staff. These programmes start from 2 weeks after discharge and allow the patient to continue to increase the exercise undertaken with the supervision and advice of health-care professionals, as well as creating a social environment conducive to recovery.

The following exercises can be encouraged.

Shoulder and girdle exercises

Big circles should be made by rolling the shoulders forwards and backwards.

Arm exercises

With the patient standing, raise both hands out to the side, then up above the head. This should be repeated 10 times.

Breathing exercises

Patients should place their hands on their chest to feel the ribs as they breathe in. Patients should take a deep breath in, hold it for 3 seconds, followed by a sigh. This should be repeated at regular intervals.

House and garden activities

The sternum usually takes about 3 months to heal and 'knit' back together. It is usual for the patient to feel a slight clicking movement of the sternum during the initial 2 weeks – the sternum is only held together by wires. It should have settled by the time the patient is reviewed at the follow-up clinic after 8–12 weeks. On occasion, a patient may have what is known as an unstable sternum, which usually requires re-wiring under a further general anaesthetic.

To prevent an unstable sternum, patients should be warned against lifting objects heavier than 10 pounds (4.5 kg) in weight and to avoid any pushing or pulling activities such as:

- using a vacuum cleaner
- carrying heavy shopping
- lifting up young children
- moving heavy furniture
- strenuous gardening.

All these activities put stress and pressure on to the chest.

Patients may still be able to undertake light household duties and gardening, such as dusting, washing light dishes, pruning and watering plants with a hosepipe or light watering can. Activity can be gradually increased, and the patient is the best judge of what he or she feels capable of. In surveys of lifestyles after surgery, the duties performed in the house appear to be the biggest adjustment made by the patient and spouse/partner. In 1997, Jickling and Graydon suggested that women used levels of fatigue and home responsibility to guide activities, in contrast to men who followed specific discharge instructions from care-givers.

Compliance with anti-embolism stockings

It is essential that time is taken to teach patients the correct method of application and how to care for the stockings. If the leg has been measured carefully, the hosiery should fit and provide appropriate graduation of pressure from the ankle to the knee. Correctly measured and applied stockings will feel comfortable and so aid compliance. Patients should be shown how to remove wrinkles and advised against folding the stockings over at the top.

Application can be made easier if rubber gloves are worn, which make the stockings easier to grip (this also protects the stockings from snagging on sharp fingernails) and moisturising the leg before putting on provides added comfort. Regular washing of the stockings prolongs their life, and provision of two pairs allows for continued use.

Driving

The sternal wound does not exempt a patient from wearing a seat belt in a car. If discomfort is felt from a seat belt, a pillow can be used between the sternum and seat belt to enhance comfort. Doctors may not be willing to provide a letter of exemption. The DVLA provides guidance on how long patients must wait after surgery before driving. This is for guidance only and is the minimal time; patients recover at different rates and so may require a longer recovery before driving (Table 11.1).

Flying

Patients can safely fly after cardiac surgery, but plans should be delayed for at least 12 weeks following the surgery. Patients going on long flights (longer than 2 hours) should be encouraged to walk at regular intervals in the aisle. If this is not possible, movement of the feet every half hour will help to prevent sluggish circulation in the legs. It may be beneficial for the patient to wear anti-embolism stockings to reduce the risk of embolism.

Hygiene and wound care

During the first couple of months patients should be encouraged to take showers rather than baths if possible. This prevents added strain and pressure on the chest wall, and will prevent 'dirty' water from contaminating healing wounds. Very hot or very cold water may also make the patient dizzy, and where feasible it should be suggested that showers or

Table 11.1 Return to driving after cardiac surgery

Operation	Group 1	Group 2
Coronary artery bypass graft	Driving must cease for 4 weeks. Driving may recommence thereafter, providing that there is no other disqualifying conditions. DVLA need not be notified	Disqualified from driving for at least 6 weeks Relicensing may be permitted there-after, provided that the exercise test requirement can be met and there is no other disqualifying condition
Pacemaker insertion	Driving must cease for 4 weeks Driving may be permitted thereafter, providing that there are no other disqualify-ing conditions. License should be subject to review at least every 3 years	Disqualified from driving for 3 months Relicensing may be permitted there-after, unless there are other disqualify-ing conditions
ICD	Driving can recur when the following criteria have been met: • The device has been implanted for 6 months and has not fired in that time • Any previous discharge must not have been accompanied by incapacity • Device is subject to regular review with interrogation • A period of 1 month off driving must elapse after revision of the device (generator or electrode) or alteration of antiarrhythmic drugs • There is no other disqualify-ing factor • The licence will be subject to annual review	Permanent bar
Heart transplant	Driving may continue provided no other disqualify-ing condition DVLA need not be notified	Disqualified from driving if symptomatic Relicensing may be permitted provided that there is no other disqualifying conditions

Table 11.1 (contd)

Operation	Group 1	Group 2
Valve disease	Driving may continue, provided no other disqualifying condition such as continued arrhythmias DVLA need not be notified	Relicensing may be permitted provided that there is no other disqualifying condition

Note that, although the DVLA may not need to be notified, it should be declared to insurance companies.
The licence holder must notify the DVLA unless otherwise stated.
Taken from At a Glance Guide to the Current Medical Standards of Fitness to Drive issued by Drivers' Medical Unit, DVLA, Swansea, March 1998.
ICD, implantable cardioverter defibrillator.

baths are taken when they are accompanied in the house. In addition patients should be encouraged to wear clean clothes after showering or bathing.

Many patients may be frightened about taking baths or showers in case the wounds become wet, but these fears are unfounded. Surgical wounds can be washed gently with soap and water without pressing hard. Areas should be patted dry so that disruption to the healing process is minimised. The natural healing process will result in flakes of tissue and skin gradually falling from the wound.

On occasion, the patient may complain of the wound being sore and itchy. It is not uncommon to observe slight swelling and redness. It is only necessary for the patient to seek help if the wound becomes hot to the touch, more reddened and inflamed, starts to ooze and becomes increasingly painful. When this happens, wounds should be assessed by a healthcare professional, and antibiotics started only if an infection is confirmed. Patients who have had coronary artery bypass grafts involving the IMA are likely to experience numbness on the side of the chest affected. This sensation will not resolve and is perfectly natural, but it is often a cause of concern for patients.

Sutures used are generally dissolvable. Occasionally a knot from the sutures may appear through the skin, and this may become troublesome to the patient because it catches on clothes or may initiate oozing around the area. This can be relieved by cutting off the knot using an aseptic technique. After coronary artery bypass grafts, it is not uncommon for leg wounds to be more troublesome than sternal wounds. Leg oedema after surgery and the need for exercise often contribute to trauma to the suture line and subsequent oozing. Studies suggest that the incidence of oozing in these wounds is as high as 75%, but it is unclear whether this incidence relates to infected wounds. With earlier discharge, some leg wounds do not ooze until after discharge.

Sexual intercourse

Research has shown that sexual intercourse does not raise the heart rate any higher than when climbing two flights of stairs. Most patients have demonstrated that they can climb the stairs with no ill-effects before discharge. Resumption of sexual intercourse is therefore individual, but the main obstruction may be chest discomfort rather than physical ability.

Medication

Patients should have verbal information about the drugs that they are taking. This information should include the reason for taking the medication, what effects the medication has, any side effects/problems that may occur, the most suitable time to take the medication and whether to take with or without food. The importance of not stopping medication unless under instructions from the doctor should be stressed. Women appear to place more importance on knowing the meaning of symptoms and side effects of medications, whereas men place importance on recovery time and lifestyle modifications (Jickling and Graydon, 1997).

Aspirin

Arterial thrombus, such as that which occurs in coronary thrombosis, results partly from an aggregation of platelets, which ultimately form plugs in blood vessels. By decreasing platelet aggregation, through the use of aspirin, this may inhibit thrombus formation in the arterial side of the circulation. All patients undergoing cardiac surgery should be started on aspirin unless they display one or more of the following contraindications:

* known hypersensitivity to aspirin
* active (i.e. symptomatic) peptic ulcer
* haemophilia and other bleeding disorders
* treatment with warfarin or other anticoagulant.

Patient compliance may be improved if they are informed that aspirin is being given for its antiplatelet properties rather than its analgesic properties. Patients should be advised to take aspirin with or after food because this will reduce the likelihood of dyspepsia. For patients who have problems with indigestion, enteric-coated aspirin is advised.

The dosage of aspirin can vary between institutions and consultants. The doses range from 75 mg to 150 mg. Some surgeons show a preference for enteric-coated aspirin regardless of any previous history of gastric irritation, whereas others reserve enteric-coated for those who demonstrate adverse effects to aspirin. Patients who are unable to tolerate aspirin in any form can be prescribed ticlopidine, and this requires 3-monthly screening of platelets.

Vasodilators

Nitrates are not usually required after cardiac surgery, although patients who have been dependent on sublingual glyceryl trinitrate (GTN) may be reluctant to stop carrying the medication. The transition is easier if education about the pain characteristics is given. Patients who have undergone bypass grafts using the radial artery as a conduit may require a course of diltiazem.

β Blockers

Patients requiring β blockers preoperatively may continue on this therapy postoperatively. A natural response to stress, excitement or emotion is the release of catecholamines, which increase the heart rate and subsequently the myocardial demands. β-adrenoceptor antagonists, e.g. atenolol, block the β actions of noradrenaline released from the cardiac sympathetic stimulation and circulating adrenaline, producing a reduction in the force and contraction of the ventricle. β blockers slow the heart rate and lower blood pressure, thereby reducing myocardial demand and myocardial workload. Abrupt withdrawal may lead to tachycardia, and to increased myocardial work and increased blood pressure. There are several known side effects:

- Patients may become more aware of dreaming
- Sex drive may be decreased
- People with diabetes may have changes in normal glucose levels and β blockers may mask the signs of hypoglycaemia.

β blockers should be used with caution and closely monitored in patients with asthma.

Anticoagulants

Warfarin is required indefinitely for patients after the following:

- mechanical valve replacement
- sustained atrial fibrillation
- prosthetic mitral valves and a large left atrium
- identified left atrial thrombus
- identified history of systemic embolisation.

Warfarin requirement for patients with tissue valves is optional if the patient remains in sinus rhythm.

Patients on anticoagulation are at risk of haemorrhage, but discontinuation of warfarin may be disastrous. The effect of warfarin is measured as the international normalised ratio (INR), which expresses the prothrombin time relative to an international standard for thromboplastin reagents. The incidence of haemorrhage is proportional to the INR. Patients receiving warfarin therapy require education to help maintain a stable INR. Not only is clotting influenced by drug interactions, it is also influenced by diet and alcohol.

After valve surgery, or for the treatment of atrial fibrillation, INR is maintained between 2.5 and 3.5 and requires regular monitoring. Results outside this range will require a further period of hospitalisation because of the risk of clotting or over-anticoagulation. Over-anticoagulation is modified most safely with fresh frozen plasma. The use of vitamin K (the antibody to warfarin) to reverse anticoagulation may make control very difficult for a long period. Insufficient anticoagulation may be corrected by increased dosages of warfarin, although there will be a time delay in effectiveness, or short-term heparin infusion with concurrent warfarin therapy may be required. Patients receiving warfarin should inform medical and dental staff of this before any procedures.

Rich food, particularly foods with a high vitamin K content, can have an effect of lowering an INR, but it does not mean that these foods are to be avoided. Alcohol potentiates the effects of warfarin and, to prevent major disruption to INRs, binge drinking should be discouraged, although regular habits in relation to diet and fluids help to stabilise blood results. Analgesics used for headaches either containing paracetamol or combined with co-proxamol are relatively safe in doses of two to four tablets a day once or twice a week, but regular ingestion of six to eight tablets daily may require a reduction in the dose of warfarin. Patients taking warfarin should carry a card to inform health professionals, at the time of emergencies, that they take anticoagulants.

Lipid-lowering drugs

Cardiac surgery does not affect cholesterol levels, and medication started preoperatively to maintain cholesterol levels within the normal range should be continued postoperatively and on discharge. It must be remembered that these drugs must be combined with a low-fat diet. For patients who are unaware of the cholesterol level, the preoperative fast before surgery is an opportune time to take a fasting lipid level. Slight elevation of cholesterol at this time may, however, be stress related, so any results must be treated with caution; they are still useful in identifying an elevated level which may require further investigation after surgery.

Antibiotic prophylaxis

Patients undergoing prosthetic valve replacement should always receive prophylactic antibiotic for further dental or surgical treatment.

Ranitidine

As a result of the potential stress response to the operating room, prophylactic oral administration of Zantac (ranitidine) can reduce the development of gastric ulceration. Some centres advocate the use of oral Zantac for 6 weeks postoperatively or longer if the patient develops complications that require a longer period on the ventilator.

Relatives

Once discharged, most patients do not require the services of the primary health-care team, so their only contact with a health-care professional may be an occasional visit to their own general practitioners to collect a repeat prescription. After discharge, most patients will not experience complications. However, a significant population will, and there is concern that carers do not always know what to do in the case of complications. It is also recognised that GPs and district nurses may not have the specialist knowledge to provide the relevant advice (Davies, 2000). It is important that, even if the patient and spouse/partner are offered the opportunity to attend formal rehabilitation, they have a number to contact if they have any worries.

An interesting study by Gillis (1984) demonstrated that patients always reported that they were happy to go home, even when the time to discharge was shortened. In contrast, partners frequently expressed fears relating to the responsibility of looking after somebody so close to major surgery. In the early period of discharge, it appears that the carers require some support, with the patient receiving support from the carer. Carers have described this early discharge period as demanding and frightening. It does appear that emphasis is placed on the role of the carer. The usual practice is to send patients home only when they have a responsible person staying with them for the first few weeks after discharge. If this is not a feasible option, patients may have a period of convalescence arranged.

A number of support groups have developed in connection with cardiac surgery or intervention. These are run by patients and can provide useful peer support for both the patient and his or her relatives.

A study by Johnson (2000) identified the main complications experienced by patients within the first 4 weeks after discharge. They fell into the seven main categories shown in Table 11.2, and 9% of patients required readmission into hospital, predominantly as a result of pleural effusions and atrial fibrillation, which are considered to be the two most commonly identified postoperative complications after cardiac surgery (Emery and Pearson, 1998). The other main complications identified by Johnson (2000) were pain, wounds, gastrointestinal disturbances and miscellaneous problems. The gastrointestinal problems were usually related to loss of appetite or nausea, common problems after surgery (Jaarma et al., 1995). Other frequently mentioned occurrences were blurred vision, hoarse voice and depression.

Table 11.2 The incidence of common complications after cardiac surgery

Problem	Percentage
Respiratory	22
Cardiac	9
Wounds	29
Gastrointestinal	13
Pain	8
Neurological	6
Miscellaneous	13

References

Barnason S, Zimmerman L, Anderson A, Mohr Burt S, Nieveen J (2000) Functional status outcome of patient with coronary artery bypass grafts over time. *Heart Lung* **29**: 33–46.

Davies N (2000) Carers' opinions and emotional responses following cardiac surgery: cardiac rehabilitation implications for critical care nurses. *Intensive Crit Care Nursing* **16**: 66–75.

Department of Health (1995) *The Health of the Nation, Key Area Handbook. Coronary Heart Disease.* London: HMSO.

Emery C, Pearson S (1998) Managing coronary artery disease. In: Shuldham C, ed., *Cardiorespiratory Nursing.* Cheltenham: Stanley Thornes, pp. 332–72.

Gillis CL (1984) Reducing family stress during and after coronary artery bypass surgery, *Nursing Clin North Am* **19**(1): 103–11.

Jaarma T, Kastermans M, Dassen T, Philipsen (1995) Problems of cardiac patients in early recovery. *J Adv Nursing* **21**: 21–7.

Jickling J, Graydon J (1997) The information needs at the time of hospital discharge of male and female patients who have undergone CABG. A pilot study. *Heart Lung* **26**: 350–7.

Johnson K (2000) Use of telephone follow-up for post-cardiac surgery patients. *Intensive Crit Care Nursing* **16**: 144–50.

Moore C (1995) A comparison of women's and men's symptoms during home recovery after coronary artery bypass surgery. *Heart Lung* **24**: 495–501.

Rowe MA, King KB (1998) Long term chest wall discomfort in women after coronary artery bypass grafts. *Heart Lung* **2**:7 184–8.

Sanchez R, Jacob I, Newark NJ (1994) Temporal relationship of complications after coronary bypass surgery: scheduling for safe discharge. *Am Heart J* **127**: 282–6.

Index